T0163202

POCKET
FIRST AID AND
WILDERNESS MEDICINE

About the authors

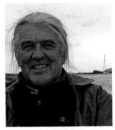

Dr Jim Duff has more than 40 years' experience of climbing, trekking, sailing and teaching wilderness medicine, first aid and leadership in the Himalayas, Australia and East Africa.

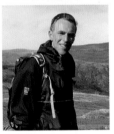

Dr Ross Anderson, a fell runner, lives on the edge of Lake District in the UK where he is a GP and enjoys free time in the mountains. He holds the UIAA Diploma in Mountain Medicine and is the medical consultant for a major trek and expedition company.

POCKET
FIRST AID AND
WILDERNESS MEDICINE

by
Dr Jim Duff MBChB, BSc
and
Dr Ross Anderson MBChB, MRCS, MRCGP

© Dr Jim Duff and Dr Ross Anderson 2017
12th edition (3rd by Cicerone) 2017
ISBN: 978 1 85284 913 9
Reprinted 2019, 2022 (with updates)

11th edition (2nd by Cicerone) 2012
10th edition (1st by Cicerone) 2007

First nine editions published by Treksafe.

Printed in Singapore by KHL Printing.
A catalogue record for this book is available from the British Library.

Artwork: Clare Crooke

To the local people who make our journeys possible.

WARNING

This book is offered to people who find themselves managing accidents or illnesses in remote situations without immediate access to medical help. It contains advanced treatments and techniques as a reminder to people who have been trained to carry them out. Do nothing above your skill level. If you are not sure or don't know it, don't do it!

Comments, suggestions and criticism are always welcome: contact the authors at info@treksafe.com.au (www.treksafe.com.au).

Front cover: Camp 2 at midnight, Western Cwm, Mount Everest, SW face (1975)

CONTENTS

ACRONYMS AND ABBREVIATIONS

AMS	acute mountain sickness
BLS	basic life support
cap	capsule (of medication)
cm	centimetre(s)
CO	carbon monoxide
CPR	cardio pulmonary resuscitation
CSMS	circulation, sensation, movement, strength
DCI	decompression illness
DRSABCS	deadly bleeding, response, send for help, airway, breathing, circulation, specific situations
ETA	estimated time of arrival
EPIRB	emergency position indicating radio beacon
g	gram(s)
HACE	high altitude cerebral edema
HAPE	high altitude pulmonary edema
IM	intramuscular
IV	intravenous
L	litres
L/min	litre(s) per minute
LLS	Lake Louise Score
LZ	landing zone
m	metre(s)
mg	milligram(s)
min	minute(s)
MOI	mechanism of injury
NSAID	non-steroidal anti-inflammatory drug
ORS	oral rehydration solution
PIB	pressure immobilization bandage
PLB	personal locator beacon
psi	pounds per square inch
SAR	search and rescue (organization)
SC	subcutaneous (under the skin)
STI	sexually transmitted infection
tab	tablet
TM	trademark (indicates a trademarked name)

CONVERSION TABLES

1 litre	1.75 pints (British), 2.1 pints (American)
2.5 cm	1 inch
1 metre	3.3 feet (39.4 inches)
1 km	0.6 mile
1 kg	2.2 pounds
1°C	1.8°F
37°C	98.6°F

Acknowledgements

Thank you to all our friends and colleagues who contributed advice. Some of them are mentioned below but there are many others, including the trek leaders and guides we trained on our courses, who gave us valuable feedback.

Dr Peter Gormly, who passed away in 2012, wrote the Australian National Antarctic Research Expeditions (ANARE) First Aid Manual and we owe a debt of gratitude to him and all who contributed to that publication.

Réjane's enduring skill and dedication brought the book into being in the first place and the inestimable staff at Cicerone have put it all together.

Special thanks to my friends and colleagues for their advice and support, namely doctors Edi Albert, Buddha Basnyat, Trish Batchelor, John Blyth, Domhnall Brannigan, Louise Cook, Renée Farrrar (dental problems), David Hillebrandt, Catherine Mangham, Nick Mason, Annemarie Newth, Prativa Pandey, Sue Partridge, Jae Spinaze, and also Lucas Trihey.

PREFACE

Venturing into remote areas on land or water involves a degree of risk. Minimizing these risks, while feeling confident in your ability to deal with any potential injury or illness, is part of the challenge and satisfaction of wilderness travel. One definition of wilderness is 'more than four hours from medical help', so even travellers in remote areas of developed countries may find themselves put to the test.

First aid is the provision of an immediate response to an accident or illness until timely medical help is available. ***Wilderness medicine*** means providing first aid, THEN continuing to treat and care for injured or ill people for an extended period of time without external help and with limited resources. Wilderness medicine requires diagnostic skills and abilities well beyond the scope of first aid.

Pocket First Aid and Wilderness Medicine sets out to provide the information needed to avoid or manage commonly occurring problems.

Part 1: The fundamentals should be read thoroughly as it covers the essentials of preparation, prevention, general care for the sick and injured, the use of medications and pain management.

Part 2: Accident and illness protocol sets out the standard procedures to follow in any accident or illness situation, including how to deal with immediate life-threatening situations. Importantly it sets out how to work out what the problem is (the diagnosis).

Part 3: Problems and their treatment covers specific accidents and illnesses.

The **Appendices** are a rich source of information, especially the chart of medications and suggested first aid kits for different groups and skill levels.

READ THIS ↓ READ THIS ↓ READ THIS ↓

- Information in this book is highly condensed: get to know the general layout and contents before you need it. Subjects are cross-referenced and indexed.
- 'Victim' is used throughout the book instead of 'patient', 'casualty' etc.
- When a treatment is described, it is assumed that a primary survey (Chapters 6 and 7), shock prevention and stabilization (Chapter 8) and secondary survey (Chapter 9) have been carried out as necessary.
- For any accident or illness there may be several ways to manage the problem: for clarity and brevity, we have chosen those we believe to be simple and effective.
- Symptoms and signs are set down roughly in order of appearance or importance. Although listed, symptoms and signs may not all appear in a given situation.
- Treatments are presented in order of preference (including antibiotics) and in the order in which they are carried out.
- Trained first aiders have a 'duty of care'. Always obtain consent and record all steps of diagnosis and treatment. Certain treatments and techniques are described as a reminder to people who have been trained to carry them out. **Make sure that you do nothing inappropriate for your skill level.**
- Certain procedures described should not be used if medical help is available within the time indicated in the text.
- Generic names of medications are used throughout the text and some common trade names are given in the chart of medications (identified with a 'TM').
- When a medication is suggested, it is to be given by mouth unless otherwise stated.
- Antibiotics are important in remote situations and their use is suggested in the text while dose and notes are in Appendix 2. Suitable levels of training are required.
- Antibiotics for particular conditions may change as resistance develops. If this book is more than three years old, check out Appendix 2 with your doctor!
- The procedures, and medications in particular, mentioned in this book are for fit healthy adults only. If you have pre-existing medical problems, consult your doctor about any possible interactions or contra-indications. Check with your doctor for children's medications and dose.
- The term 'hyperbaric bag' is used instead of 'portable hyperbaric chamber', 'pressure bag', 'Gamow bag' or their trade names (PAC™, Certec™, Gamow™).

1. PREVENTION

Preparation (hope for the best, plan for the worst)

In general

- Trips should be chosen to suit the level of fitness and expertise of the weakest member of your group.
- Check that your equipment is in good condition and suitable for the area and for the worst conditions you may meet.
- Allow three months for all major overseas pre-trip preparations. Arrange for your vaccinations plus a medical and dental examination. Pre-existing medical conditions should be thoroughly checked by a doctor who understands the environment you intend to visit.
- Those with pre-existing illnesses must bring enough of their regular medication for the whole trip, and pack a reserve supply separately. Check whether it is heat sensitive and whether it will work under the conditions expected; ask your doctor/pharmacist whether any of it will interact with the drugs in your first aid kit. Those with allergies to specific medications must bring alternatives.
- You will need travel insurance, making sure it covers emergency evacuation, by helicopter if necessary, and your specific activity (eg diving). In many countries, proof of your ability to pay (insurance cover, credit card number or cash) is needed for prompt emergency air evacuation. Leave a copy of your insurance with your travel agent, trek company and/or embassy along with a copy of your passport and details of next-of-kin.
- **Travelling with controlled drugs/medications** (opiates, ketamine, even codeine) may be illegal in some countries, even in transit, so you MUST carry appropriate customs forms and your doctor's letter/prescription. Check country requirements with your travel agent, pharmacist, doctor, consulate or embassy (see Appendix 10 – 'Travel Medicine and General Information').
- There are many serious infectious diseases worldwide, most of them occurring in tropical or subtropical zones. Owing to global warming, the range of many diseases is spreading. Research and preparation before leaving home are essential and vaccination/prevention is much better than treatment: see 'Keeping healthy', p. 14.
- For any trip, however short and easy, leave details of your intended route and estimated time of arrival (ETA) with a reliable person or the relevant organization (and remember to let them know once you're safe!).

- Carry maps, GPS, mobile/satellite phone and/or radio (VHF or HF) and a personal locator beacon (PLB) or EPIRB, as appropriate. See 'Good Communication', p. 79.

Children

Children deteriorate more quickly than adults when ill or injured, and they are more susceptible than adults to hypothermia, heat exhaustion and dehydration. If a child has lost consciousness, however briefly, they should be evacuated (exception: an obvious case of simple faint). Between ages 4 to 7 years, children become increasingly able to tell you reasonably clearly what they are feeling. Below age 4, the only signs that a child is developing a serious illness may be increased fussiness, crying, loss of interest or appetite, or becoming quiet, drowsy or unresponsive.

Risks in pregnancy

The *relatively* safer time to travel is during the middle three months of a pregnancy, but risks still include miscarriage, life-threatening bleeding, tubal (ectopic) pregnancy and premature labour. Infections that can damage the foetus (especially malaria, rubella, Zika, hepatitis A and E) are a possibility.

- As a general rule, do not ascend above 2500m during pregnancy and avoid high-risk malarial areas and scuba-diving. See 'Childbirth in a wilderness setting', p. 196, and 'Pregnancy', p. 38.

Notes for group leaders/doctors

Your position brings with it a professional duty of care and you must understand the ramifications of this thoroughly.

- Research the area you are going to: note the locations and phone details of hospitals, clinics and rescue organizations, means of communication and evacuation.
- It is your responsibility to see that water, food, kitchens and toilets are appropriate and sanitary.
- Before departure speak to all participants and check their insurance cover, passport and next-of-kin details (keeping copies). Instruct them to get as fit as possible. Ask about their health. If they have a pre-existing medical problem, they should see a doctor about the intended trip: have them explain to you how to deal with possible emergencies (eg testing a diabetic's blood sugar level, dealing with an asthma attack).
- On the trip, give daily (or more frequent) briefings to your group and staff on what to expect on the next stage of the trip.

- Put the **buddy system** in place: pair everyone up with instructions to keep a careful eye on each other in order to detect early signs of illness or other problems as soon as possible (see box below). Buddies must tell the leader/doctor of their suspicions immediately (preferably without telling their sick partner, who will often minimize or deny problems). Leaders, doctors and first aiders must also have a buddy.
- As the doctor/leader, you should briefly check every member of the group morning, noon and night. Early detection of problems needs an appreciation of the terrain to be covered and of potential environmentally-induced problems. Have a high index of suspicion and a readiness to act promptly.
- If you are worried that someone is becoming unwell, stop as soon as it is safe to do so and carefully look into the problem.
- Hypothermia, dehydration, low blood sugar (due to lack of food), altitude illness and exhaustion are common in the wilderness setting. They share some similar symptoms and signs, and may occur together. If one condition is found, check for the others and check the whole group.

EARLY NON-SPECIFIC SIGNS OF SOMEONE BECOMING UNWELL (easily remembered as the 'umbles':
grumble, mumble, bumble, fumble, stumble)

Changes are more significant when they are 'out of character'.

- Personality changes: anxiety, irritability, anger, excitability, complaining, depression, loss of concentration, making poor decisions
- Behavioural changes: tiredness, lethargy, coming to camp late and last, social withdrawal, going to bed early and being last to get out of bed, disturbed sleep, loss of appetite, missing meals
- Clumsiness, staggering, falling over, dropping things, inability to tie shoelaces or pack own bag etc

Keeping healthy

Preventing diarrhoea and food poisoning
Attention to detail dramatically reduces the incidence of these common scourges.

- Disinfect all drinking water (see below).

DISINFECTING WATER TO MAKE IT SAFELY DRINKABLE

Disinfecting water is making it safely drinkable, ie free enough of germs (viruses, bacteria, protozoa) that cause diarrhoea and other infectious diseases. Select the cleanest/clearest water from the best possible site (eg above village/campsite rather than below it, running rather than still). Disinfection methods include heat, filtration, chemicals, UV (ultra-violet) light, distillation (solar stills). Combining methods increases the desired effect. See UIAA advice on 'Water disinfection' in Appendix 10.

Method 1: boil water till bubbling commences. This is sufficient what-ever the altitude. **Note:** boiling is the only way to disinfect water con-taminated with cyclospora, but does not kill Hep A (protection is only guaranteed by vaccination).

Method 2: filtration. Use a good quality filter and preferably combine with one other form of disinfection (boiling, chemical or UV). In an emergency use layers of sand and charcoal in a waterproof bag with a hole in the bottom. Cloudy, dirty water should be allowed to settle, then filtered.

Method 3: adding a chemical

1. Chlorine as hypochlorite or NaDCC tablets: follow the instructions carefully.

In an emergency you can use unscented household bleach (5% hypochlorite solution – check the concentration on the bottle): add 2 drops per litre (there are approximately 70 drops in a teaspoon) and shake well. Wait 30 minutes. The water should now smell faintly of chlorine. If it does not, add 2 more drops per litre. **Note:** once a bottle is opened, bleach loses its potency after six months.

2. Iodine tablets: follow instructions, best used for short duration as can affect thyroid gland. In an emergency use povi-iodine (6 drops/litre), wait one hour. To get rid of any chemical taste, add a small amount of vitamin C or other flavour after the wait time is up.

Note: the longer you leave the chemical treatments, the more effec-tive they are. At least double the waiting times for very polluted, cloudy or cold water.

4: UV light eg SteriPEN™: They are battery driven (carry spares), need gentle agitation while in operation, have reduced efficiency in cloudy water (filter first) and are fragile so carry an alternative method. In an emergency use the sun's UV light: expose water in a clear plastic bottle to six hours of sunlight or three days in cloudy conditions.

- Avoid touching your mouth with your hands ('buddies' can remind each other).
- Wash hands frequently and thoroughly (45 seconds) with soap and water (alcohol wipes/sanitizer gels are an aid, not a substitute for soap and water). Then dry them thoroughly with a clean towel, or air dry (drying is as important as washing). This is especially important if working in the kitchen, and after each bowel motion/visit to a toilet (toilets must be fly proof).
- No one with diarrhoea (or other infectious diseases) should be allowed near food preparation, serving or washing up.
- All kitchen utensils must be kept scrupulously clean. Cooks must have two chopping boards and knives: one set for preparing meat and fish only (this set must be thoroughly washed and scalded after every use), and one for all other purposes. Keep flies, cockroaches and rats off prepared food and preparation surfaces.
- Vegetables should be well cooked, or washed and soaked in chemical solution for at least one hour (use double the recommended dose of chemical for method 3 of water disinfection, below). However carefully prepared, salads may still cause diarrhoea.
- Peel fruit, boil fresh milk. Avoid curd, lassi, milk shakes, ice cream, local honey and home brewed beer.
- All cooked food should be eaten immediately. Avoid reheated food (if this cannot be avoided, reheat thoroughly to *reduce* the risk).

Preventing spread of infection
- Anyone suffering from an infectious/contagious disease (such as diarrhoea, hepatitis, eye/wound infection, meningitis, pneumonia, influenza, measles or chickenpox) should be 'quarantined'. Check your group, including staff, for any sign of the illness.
- Ideally, isolate the victim in a room or tent on their own, keeping their dishes, cutlery, soap and towel separate.
- Help the victim to keep good personal hygiene.
- Wear protective/rubber gloves when attending the victim, especially when cleaning up blood, vomit or stools.
- Carer and victim should wear face masks (improvised if necessary) in

cases of meningitis, pneumonia, influenza etc. This is especially important if the victim is coughing or sneezing.
- Wear gloves and goggles (or sunglasses) when treating wounds (to protect from blood-borne viruses – eg hepatitis B and C, HIV), especially when jet washing them.
- Wash and carefully dry hands after contact with the victim, their clothes or belongings.

Preventing animal and insect bites/stings
- Do not approach animals too closely. Do not surprise, feed or pet them.
- All animal (and human!) bites should be treated very thoroughly as they are likely to become infected.
- **Dogs, monkeys, bats and foxes** and many other animals may bite, causing injuries or infection (including tetanus and rabies). While most animals are likely to bite when they are surprised, injured or already fighting, rabid animals often attack without cause and they often bite more than once, or more than one person. Rabid dogs may appear aggressive, carry their tails between their legs, and salivate or foam at the mouth; their eyes may be red. They usually die within 10 days. However, there may be none of these signs. Pre-exposure rabies vaccination is available and is recommended for long-term travellers, residents or those at special risk (even vaccinated people will still need a post exposure course of treatment if bitten).
- **Bears:** polar bears are the most dangerous, closely followed by grizzly (brown) bears. Most bear attacks occur when bears are surprised, have young, have lost their natural fear of humans, or are old or injured. Food and all other smelly items including food waste should be stashed 100m away from campsites which should be in open country. The camp and yourself must be meticulously clean and odour free (this includes soap etc). Travel in groups of four or more, carry a bear spray, make noise, avoid dense foliage and walking at night. If confronted, freeze, no eye contact, talk in low reassuring tones and slowly back off. Do not run or climb trees. If charged, use bear spray. If savaged by a brown bear: play dead, face down, hands over neck. If savaged by a black bear: fight back.
- **Sharks and crocodiles:** attacks are rare worldwide but more common in certain areas. Sharks congregate around seal colonies and migrating whales, and they may travel long distances up rivers. They feed mainly in the early morning or late evening. If approached, face it and back slowly away. If charged, assume the cold water survival position. If bitten, attack the eyes, gills and snout. Divers may seek shelter on the bottom,

swimmers against rocks, reef or jetty piles

Crocodiles inhabit warmer rivers and estuaries and saltwater crocodiles may travel hundreds of kilometres out to sea from their estuarine breeding grounds. They are territorial stealth hunters. Camping, wading or swimming in areas where they live is not recommended. Ocean beaches well away from a river mouth are considered to be safer. Consult knowledgeable locals.

- **Snakes, spiders and scorpions:** do not reach into holes, avoid climbing on vegetated rock or swimming from dense foliage on the shore, be wary when moving rocks or collecting firewood. Use a torch at night. Check inside your kayak, raft, sleeping bag and tent (keep it zipped up) before getting in. Check clothes and boots before putting them on. Wear long trousers, gaiters, boots and gloves. Scorpions are attracted to condensation under groundsheets. Wear strong footwear when wading on coral or in murky water. **Note:** carry the equivalent of two 15cm elastic or crepe bandages which is the minimum necessary to put a pressure immobilization bandage (PIB) on a leg (see 'Pressure immobilization bandage (PIB)', p. 125).
- **Jellyfish stings:** for prevention wear a full body Lycra™ stinger suit.

Preventing mosquito-borne diseases

Mosquitoes may carry serious diseases such as malaria, dengue fever, Japanese encephalitis, Ross River fever, yellow fever, West Nile disease or Zika virus. Avoiding mosquito bites is a vital first-line defence against these fearsome diseases.

- Use personal repellent containing DEET (20–50%), applied *over* sunscreens. Use sprays, heated repellent tablets and/or mosquito coils in your rooms on arrival (including the bathroom) and at night.
- In the evening and night, wear long sleeves, trousers and socks sprayed with repellent and/or permethrin.
- Sleep under an undamaged mosquito net (coated with permethrin for extra effectiveness), tucked under your mattress.
- Preventative medications for **malaria**: seek travel medicine advice before setting off as drug-resistant strains of malaria are common. These drugs need to be started before entering the malarial zone and continued for some time afterwards. They do not guarantee full protection and may have side effects such as rashes, nausea, dizziness, diarrhoea, increased risk of sunburn, vivid dreams and severe mental disturbance (the latter especially with mefloquine). Side effects often appear or seem to get worse at altitude.
- Avoid scuba-diving while taking malaria medications.

- If you have had malaria before, or are going to a remote malarial area with no medical help, carry a supply of treatment medication (eg Riamet™) and a malaria self-test kit with instructions.

Preventing other insect-borne diseases

- **Tick-borne diseases:** ticks are found in marshes, scrub, woodland, mountain meadows and deserts worldwide. Ticks carry a wide range of nasty diseases that can affect humans. To keep ticks off your skin wear long-sleeve shirts; tuck long trousers into socks and gaiters, and apply insect repellent to them. Inspect your skin (especially the hairy areas) and clothing carefully, at least 12-hourly. Shower and scrub down after possible exposure and buddy up for inspections.
- **Schistosomiasis** occurs in parts of China, South Philippines, South America and Africa (especially Lake Malawi) and is caused by a tiny skin-penetrating worm found in fresh water. Infection typically causes a brief rash followed later by a feverish illness and, later still, abdominal and bladder problems. Avoid swimming and wading in fresh water in endemic areas. Local advice on water safety may be incorrect.
- **Strongyloides** and **hookworm** are common in rural, tropical areas of Southeast Asia (including tropical Australia), Africa and South America. They are found in the soil and penetrate the skin of the feet. They can cause serious, chronic illness. Do not go barefoot on damp, bare earth in these regions, especially near villages with poor sanitation.
- **Chagas' disease** occurs in Central and South America and is caused by a beetle-like insect. Use a permethrin-soaked netting over your bed, well tucked under the mattress, when sleeping in mud, thatch or adobe houses.
- **River blindness** (tropical Central America and Africa) and **sleeping sickness** (tropical sub-Saharan Africa) are both transmitted by fly bites. Prevention is as for mosquitoes, but note that flies bite in the daytime as well.
- **Leishmaniasis** (Amazonia and Africa) is transmitted by sandfly bites. Avoid bites.

Dental problems

The best way to avoid any problems is to brush twice a day with toothpaste (preferably with fluoride), floss and avoid sugary food/drinks before bed.

Skin problems

- Protect your skin from sun, cold and wind, and do not wash with soap too frequently.

- Prevent and treat chafing, wear well-washed, well-rinsed soft under-pants/singlets. Wash, dry and powder the skin with talcum powder, or apply Vaseline™ (petroleum jelly).
- Feet may suffer blisters, fungal infections and trench foot. At the first sign of **chafing** (hot spots) apply a protective dressing and keep feet and socks warm and dry.

Deep vein thrombosis (DVT)

Prolonged lack of movement of the lower limbs (due to illness, being storm-bound, long-haul flights etc) predisposes to clots in the internal lower leg veins (DVT). Other predisposing factors include dehydration, tight clothes, bandages, splints, smoking, very high altitude and oral contraception (avoid for longer stays above 5000m and during climbs above 6000m).

- Keep your lower limbs moving on long journeys or while confined to bed/sleeping bag (point your toes at your nose then away, sets of 25 every 15 minutes). Consider compression stockings. See 'Deep vein thrombosis (DVT) and pulmonary embolus (PE)', p. 202.

Carbon monoxide (CO) poisoning

This silent killer is best prevented. In enclosed spaces with a naked flame or near an engine exhaust, assume any unexplained headache, lethargy or drowsiness is due to CO poisoning. If you can smell exhaust fumes, you are inhaling CO (but CO itself does not smell). Flames that change colour, start to flicker or go out suddenly mean that CO levels are rising dangerously.

- Ensure *good ventilation* in any shelter, snow hole, tent, boat or vehicle where there is a source of combustion (such as engines, fuel heaters, cookers, generators or lighting).
- Do not leave anything burning in confined sleeping areas.

Safety in extreme climates

Campsites

Choose campsites carefully; position pit toilets with safe access at least 30m from watercourses. Mark out a safe area on glaciers, having first probed for crevasses. Be aware of avalanche dangers, animal and insect hazards. Is there potential for flash flooding (ie canyon floors, water channels)? Seek shade or sun, depending on climate, and be aware of local ownership/feelings. Remove all rubbish.

Cold or bad weather

May cause hypothermia, frostbite or frostnip. The group or individuals may become lost or separated. Hypothermia is most likely to occur when *wind* intensifies *cold* and *wet* conditions (wet clothes lose their insulating effect). The air temperature does not have to be below freezing for hypothermia to occur. Shivering and/or the 'umbles' (see 'Notes for group leaders/doctors', p. 13) are often early signs of hypothermia and a call to act! High altitude makes hypothermia (and frostbite) more likely and more severe.

Note: for every 300m of ascent, the temperature falls about 2°C.

- Remember that it is easier to stay warm than to re-warm.
- Check forecasts and keep a weather eye open; turn back or delay departure if severe weather threatens.
- Keep your group together and check everyone regularly, remind everyone to buddy up, including local staff/porters. Be prepared to stop and shelter.
- Porters, children and old, sick, unfit, hungry or exhausted people are more likely to develop a cold injury. If one person suffers from hypothermia or frostbite, check the whole group.
- Avoid sweating and/or change wet or damp clothes for dry ones (especially gloves, socks and hat); put on warm windproof clothes before getting cold (ie *before* shivering); wear a scarf or face mask.
- Make sure footwear is not too tight, use plastic bags inside leaky footwear to keep the feet dry (paper around the toes is a good emergency insulator), use mittens rather than fingered gloves in extreme conditions and tie them to each other with string looped around the neck.
- Stop regularly and make sure everyone drinks and eats (sweets, chocolate, energy bars).
- Stop immediately and re-warm any part that goes numb (buddies often notice their partner's frostnip first).
- In sub-zero temperatures, skin may stick to metal and fuel becomes super-cooled (avoid spilling on skin).

Snow

Risks include getting lost in whiteouts, avalanche, snow blindness and loss of a ski (use leg ropes).

- The strongest people should break trail, leave someone responsible in the rear to prevent anyone getting left behind. Stop regularly to bunch up.
- Beware of avalanche slopes, especially after heavy snow falls or high winds after new snow. Heed avalanche warnings, stay on piste and open trails, spread out if you have to cross potential avalanche slopes, and

wear transceivers (inside clothing). If searching for avalanche survivors, location methods include searching for visible persons or equipment (ski poles), calling out, probing and transceivers. See Appendix 4.

- If you do have to leave a shelter in a whiteout, use a rope tied to your shelter to guide you back.
- To make crude snow gaiters and keep your socks dry, use plastic bags over your socks inside your footwear, then tape the bag over your trousers.
- Tie a strip of cloth or rope around your footwear if slipping is a problem.
- Prevent snow blindness by wearing sunglasses/goggles (wrap-around or side-shielded) at all times when at altitude and among snow and ice fields, even on cloudy days. Use a neck cord to prevent loss. If you have no sunglasses/goggles, cut slits or poke tiny holes in a piece of cardboard and tie or tape in place.

EMERGENCY SHELTERS

If you have to stop in an exposed position, especially overnight, shelter is vital. Find a place out of the wind, keep everyone together, wear all spare clothes, arrange ground insulation, eat and drink. At all times try to stay as dry as possible. Emergency snow shelters need practice and take time to construct. In an enclosed space maintain ventilation, especially if carbon monoxide poisoning is possible.

- **Bivvy/bothy bags:** improvise using a large, strong plastic bag, cutting off a corner as a breathing hole, pull the bag over your head and tuck under your body, with feet and legs in your rucksack – you will get wet in this bag through condensation.

- **'Penguin huddle':** a very effective method of maintaining body heat when a group is forced to stop in exposed conditions. Hold a tarp over the huddle to increase its effectiveness.

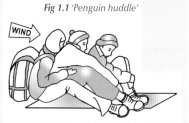

Fig 1.1 'Penguin huddle'

- **'Tibetan tuck':** a dry land version of the survival position in water, used when alone. Kneel down on a pad of insulating material. Put your rucksack to windward and tuck your head and hands around your knees.

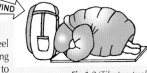

Fig 1.2 'Tibetan tuck'

- **Snow mound shelter** (snow depth <1m): pile up rucksacks, gear and branches and cover with a tarpaulin. Heap half a metre of snow onto your pile and pat down firmly. Now make an opening and extract the rucksacks, leaving an instant shelter (construction time: 2–3 hours).

- **Snow trench** (snow depth >1.5m): dig a trench and roof it with branches, tarp and snow. On a steep slope dig horizontally to form a sheltered ledge (construction time: 1–2 hours).

- **Snow hole/cave** (snow depth >2m): dig horizontally into a snow bank to make a small entrance/large cave (construction time: 2–3 hours).

At high altitude

Above 2500m, altitude illness (AMS, HACE and HAPE) becomes a possibility. Once above this altitude, a rough guide to acceptable height gain between *sleeping* altitudes is 300m per day, OR 500m per day with a rest day after every 1500m of ascent. Even these ascent rates may be too fast for some slow acclimatizers.

- Use the buddy system to detect symptoms and signs of altitude illness and check your group regularly.
- Avoid over-exertion and breathlessness while acclimatizing, especially if experiencing symptoms of AMS.
- Dehydration does not cause altitude illness, but it is an unnecessary complication. Drink enough liquid to keep your urine pale and plentiful, passing at least one litre/day. An increased urine output after an ascent is a good sign, while a decrease in urine output indicates that altitude illness (or dehydration) is developing.

- Some medications can have adverse effects at altitude.
- If you must fly or drive rapidly to 3000m or higher, spend a minimum of two nights at your arrival altitude (or lower if possible) – or until symptoms disappear – before ascending further. Consider using acetazolamide (Diamox™), especially if you have to be very active on arrival (eg group leaders, rescue personnel).

Note: coca and gingko biloba are unreliable for prevention of altitude illness. See also 'At altitude', p. 38.

Sun and wind

Sun and wind may cause burns and dehydration: extra care is needed in high, dry, cold or hot regions, and on snow or water. Apply protection (zinc oxide) to lips and nose and sunscreen to exposed areas, and wear a hat with a wide brim and maybe a scarf across your face and neck.

Hot weather

Dehydration and hot weather problems are possibilities (*heat exhaustion* is common and *heat stroke* deadly). Acclimatization to a hot climate can take up to two weeks, although two weeks of pre-departure sweating exercise in warm clothes helps. Predisposing factors to hot weather problems include fever, diarrhoea, unfitness, being overweight, youth, old age, alcohol and caffeine, and some medications (eg diuretics, beta-blockers, antihistamines, prochlorperazine/Stemetil™).

- Wear light-coloured clothing (cotton in dry climates, wicking technical wear in humid) and a broad brimmed hat/umbrella.
- Travel in the cool part of the day or at night.
- Keep your urine 'pale and plentiful', passing at least one litre/day (you may need to drink up to 1 litre/hour in very hot, dry desert conditions). As thirst is not a reliable indication of when and how much to drink, discipline yourself and your group to stop and drink regularly (at least every hour). Make drinks more attractive by adding flavour. If food and snacks are taken regularly, plain water is sufficient. If no food is being eaten, add a pinch of salt (a half teaspoon per litre) or use half strength ORS or a sports drink (see 'Dilutional (exertional) hyponatraemia (water intoxication)', p. 142).
- During heavy sweating in hot weather, especially if little food is being eaten, prevent heat cramps by adding a half teaspoon of salt to each litre of drinking water.

Lightning strike

A lightning strike may cause death (by stopping the heart), unconsciousness, severe burns (which may be internal) or blunt trauma due to being tossed or from the shock wave. When a lightning storm approaches:

- shelter in a building or vehicle with windows closed
- try not to be the highest point in the landscape
- avoid wire fences, erected tent poles (if caught in a tent, insulate yourself from the ground and don't touch the poles or ground): lay walking poles, ice axes flat on the ground
- move 50m from lightning attractors such as ridges, summits, shallow caves or cracks in rock faces, tall trees, masts or pylons
- if you are on the water, head for the shore and move at least 50m away from the water
- if you are on a via ferrata, move to a safe place where you can detach yourself from the cable
- if you are caught in the open with no shelter, spread your group out (more than 10m apart), assume the Tibetan tuck position with insulation (closed cell sleeping mat, inflatable mattress) under you and avoid touching the ground with hands or arms.

Particular situations

When taking part in any wilderness activity, the appropriate equipment (lifejackets, helmets, harnesses and technical equipment etc) should be worn/carried, and be thoroughly inspected before departure.

In the mountains

Crossing passes and *summit days:* may pose problems due to altitude, tiredness, falls, separation, cold or hot weather problems.

- When planning, consider the abilities of the weakest/slowest members and local staff (including porters).
- Keep an eye on your buddy, companions and local staff.
- Start early, maintain communication between front and rear of the group, bunch up in bad weather.
- Do not climb higher in worsening weather.

Glacier crossing: may pose problems due to hidden crevasses, falls and snow blindness. 'Dry' glaciers with no snow cover often have glacial streams (drowning and hypothermia).

- Avoid glaciers unless you have mountain skills (eg ability to perform

25

crevasse rescue) and the necessary technical equipment (crampons, ice axes, ropes, harnesses etc).

Glacial moraine walls: increase the risk of stone falls and falling into crevasses.
- Avoid if possible. Keep together or descend one at a time, or descend/ascend on a diagonal line.

Avalanche risk: increases in springtime, after midday, and during or after heavy falls of snow or rain. Villages are usually situated in avalanche-free zones, but deforestation and new settlements may not guarantee this. If villagers abandon their village, leave with them!
- Specialist skills are needed to spot and reduce avalanche dangers. Cross potential avalanche slopes only if you must, one at a time and very early in the morning.

In the desert
Losing one's way and getting lost is all too easy and help may be delayed owing to distance and poor communications. Heat and cold pose risks, and heavy rains may lead to flash flooding or vehicles bogging down in mud or soft sand. Do not head into the desert if rain is forecast! Carry enough extra water to allow a minimum of one week's survival on top of the time you expect to take.
- Check engine hoses, belts, tyres and spares before leaving. Carry sufficient spare fuel.
- Stay on tracks; note your direction and distance travelled and log your GPS positions.
- Rest in the hot part of the day to conserve energy and water.
- If lost or stuck, *stop and stay put, especially with your vehicle.* Mark your position (eg smoke, flashing mirrors, space blanket, spread-out bedding).

In the water
- If someone is in difficulty and in danger of drowning, only swim to them if you are a powerful, confident swimmer fully skilled in water rescues. Otherwise *reach* with a stick, *throw* a rope or flotation, *wait* for the current to bring them into shallow water, or *tow* them to safety.
- If you fall into cold water, the **cold water shock response** will kick in for one to three minutes, causing gasping and rapid heartbeat. Keep your head out of the water until the gasping reflex settles, as inhaling water at

this point can drown you. This response is more pronounced the colder the water, and can stop the heart. If you survive this stage, curl up into the **cold water survival position** to minimize heat loss. If you are in a group, huddle tightly together. Swimming increases the rate of heat loss, so only try to swim ashore if it is near or there is no chance of rescue.

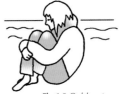

Fig 1.3 Cold water survival position

- If the water temperature is above 25°C survival time is indefinite; below this temperature hypothermia eventually causes death. Without a life jacket, the survival time in water at 10°C is 90 minutes. In near-freezing water, survival time is 10 minutes (the limbs then seize up with cold and drowning occurs); with a lifejacket the victim will stay conscious for an hour. See 'Hypothermia', p. 132.

Falling through ice: once the cold water shock response wears off, get back to where you fell in and, with arms on the ice, kick your legs to the surface and haul out. Crawl or roll away to firmer ice.

River crossings are dangerous due to the risk of drowning, injury from falls, being swept downstream and hypothermia. Check upstream and downstream for the best crossing place. Crossing alone is especially dangerous.
- Glacial streams are lower in the morning.
- Undo the waist strap of your pack (so you can discard the pack if swept away, although once off your back it can provide valuable flotation).
- Use a crossing technique (eg link arms with each other, form a circle, use a rope or pole).
- If you are swept away, try to go feet first and wait until you are swept near to the bank, or swim strongly across the current.

Surf risks include drowning or severe injury due to being 'dumped' hard on the bottom. A *rip* occurs when seawater building up against the shore flows out to sea in a strong narrow current where the waves are NOT breaking.
- Check for rips before entering the water: the outflowing rip current smoothens the surf and looks enticingly calm and green. Remember:

'Green is mean, white is right'. If caught in a rip swim across it: don't try to swim against it. Only swim for the shore once you are well to one side of the rip zone. Try not to panic! If you need help, raise an arm.
- Don't swim in waves that are breaking abruptly (dumping) on steep shores.

Water travel presents risks due to worsening weather, which can change a manageable situation abruptly, plus the danger of hypothermia and drowning.
- Lifejackets, flares, means of communications, charts, weather forecasts, proper equipment (dry/wet suits) and appropriate skills are vital. See Appendix 10 – 'Water'.

White water poses extra risks of being swept away, trapped in a rotor or foot jam.
- Equipment should include: spare paddle, helmet, harness and extraction equipment. See Appendix 10 – 'Rescue for River Runners'.

Diving: risk of hypothermia, decompression illness (DCI – including 'the bends'), nitrogen narcosis and barotrauma.
- Do not dive if unfit, obese, drunk, pregnant or suffering from epilepsy, asthma, diabetes, middle ear disease, heart disease, respiratory tract infection (especially sinusitis) or perforated ear drum or if taking medication for mental illness or malaria.
- Exertion and hypothermia predispose the diver to DCI.
- Follow dive timetables rigorously and always dive with a 'buddy'.
- Allow 24 hours after last dive before flying.

Seasickness can render a person incapable of looking after themselves, others or the boat. They may suffer dehydration and hypothermia. People prone to seasickness should take full preventive measures:
- no alcohol or strong spicy foods for 24 hours before sailing
- prepare food for a couple of days before setting off to minimize cooking
- set off in daylight and in good weather
- take an antinauseant, eg cinnarizine, Scopolamine™ patch or promethazine (Phenergan™), before symptoms start. (**Note:** promethazine induces drowsiness)
- stay on deck and steer, or go below and lie down for the first few days of a passage
- keep drinking and eating dry food (eg plain biscuits) regularly, and meals as available.

SEARCHING FOR A LOST PERSON

If one of your team is lost, stop and think carefully.

- What is their age, fitness, gear and clothing and how does this relate to weather conditions in terms of survival times, onset of hypothermia, dehydration etc?

- What was the last known location of the person and what was the time?

- Have any of their gear, clothing, footprints etc been found? If so this may help determine their speed and direction of travel.

- Are there any boundaries such as trails roads or rivers which may contain the lost person (lost people rarely cross trails or roads but tend to follow them). Note that lost people tend to gravitate downward into valleys, gullies or creeks.

- Are there any natural choke points such as bridges, passes?

- Having thought all this through, the best option for finding the person quickly is a hasty search.

- The most experienced and well equipped people available rapidly search the most likely trails and areas in teams of two. Others may be posted at choke points, to patrol boundary trails or set up a base camp.

- Use the 'call and listen' technique: stop at intervals and call the lost person's name in a loud shout, with your group waiting quietly listen for a few seconds after each call.

Time of day

End of the day: increased risk owing to fatigue, tiredness and problems due to descent, darkness etc.

- Take frequent short stops to eat, drink and rest. Take care placing your feet; increase concentration. Help exhausted people before they fall, see 'Means of evacuation', p. 79.

29

Night time: risk of getting lost or falling (leaving shelter for toilet needs has caused many injuries and deaths).
- Check toilet arrangements before dark or, better still, use a pee bottle at night (women can use a Sani-fem™ – a funnel and tube – and a pee bottle, or a good wide-mouth sealable container).

Care of local people

Porters and staff
The International Porter Protection Group (www.ippg.net) suggests the following guidelines.
- Clothing appropriate to season and altitude must be provided to porters for protection from cold, rain and snow. This may mean: windproof jacket and trousers, fleece jacket, long johns, suitable footwear (leather boots in snow), socks, hat, gloves and sunglasses.
- Above the tree line, porters should have a dedicated shelter, either a room in a lodge or a tent (the trekkers' mess tent is no good as it is not available until late evening), a sleeping pad and a blanket (or sleeping bag). They should be provided with food and warm drinks, or cooking equipment and fuel.
- Porters should be provided with the same standard of medical care that you would expect for yourself.
- The person in charge of the porters should be told to let the trek leader/ trekkers know if a porter is ill or injured, so that their condition can be assessed carefully. Failure to do this has resulted in many deaths. Ill or injured porters should never be sent down alone, but with someone who speaks their language and understands the problem, along with a letter describing their complaint. Sufficient funds should be provided to cover the cost of rescue and treatment.
- No porter should be asked to carry a load that is too heavy for their physical abilities (legal – but hardly logical – maximum weights are 20kg on Kilimanjaro, 25kg in Peru and Pakistan and 30kg in Nepal). Weight limits may need to be adjusted for altitude, trail and weather conditions: experience is needed to make this decision and to resist the local leader or sirdar's temptation to overload.

Treating local people in developing countries

While travelling in remote areas of developing countries it can be difficult to decide when to treat local people who ask you for treatment. If there is no health worker in the area for you to refer them to, consider giving help if:

- it is an emergency such as a burn, wound, broken bone or an acute severe infection
- you will be around long enough to see the treatment through
- you can provide a complete course of treatment.

In cases of chronic illness (TB, malaria, osteomyelitis etc), it is usually more appropriate to send the person to their nearest health facility with a letter noting your findings and diagnosis. If you want to do more, consider helping with payment for treatment.

2. POSITIONING AND MOVING A VICTIM

When someone is injured or ill there are certain ways to position them and specific techniques to move them that improve outcomes and reduce the risk of further injury or shock.

If the victim is likely to be in the same position for a prolonged period of time, prevent **pressure sores** by adjusting their position, if possible, every hour or two.

Positioning an accident victim

'Position found'

When a significant traumatic injury (due to a fall, rock fall, avalanche, vehicle accident etc) has occurred, initially keep the victim still in the position you find them. Moving them without examination/diagnosis and treatment (eg applying a splint) may cause shock or further injury.

Only move the victim, or their limbs, if:

- the situation is dangerous and you need to move them (and yourself) rapidly to safety
- you need access to control a life-threatening bleeding, or to their airway
- you need to turn the unconscious/semiconscious victim into the safe airway position (below)
- their position is aggravating their injuries
- uninjured limbs can be moved into a comfortable 'neutral' position
- you have completed the primary and secondary survey, and applied the necessary treatments (eg stopped bleeding, splinted broken limbs, excluded spinal injury).

Any movement should be as gentle and well thought out as time allows, using spinal immobilization techniques (see below) if appropriate.

Safe airway position

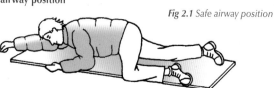

Fig 2.1 Safe airway position

This position (also called the lateral, recovery, stable side or coma position) is the best position for an unconscious or semiconscious victim who is breathing normally. It keeps the victim's airway open and free from obstruction by encouraging food, liquid, vomit, mucus or foreign objects to drain or fall from their mouth. It also prevents their tongue from obstructing their airway. Use this position if the victim is bleeding from facial or mouth injuries, even if they are fully conscious.

Nursing positions

There are positions for specific illnesses or injuries and they should make the victim feel more comfortable; check with the victim that this is so.

- **Shoulder or collar bone injury:** sitting straight up.
- **Spinal, head, pelvic injuries or fractures to one or both legs:** lying flat.
- **Difficulty breathing:** sitting up, arms on a table or semi-reclining. If breathing still remains difficult try turning or tilting the victim to one side or the other.
- **Abdominal injury:** semi-reclining, with knees raised slightly (place some support under the victim's knees).

Immobilization techniques

These are used to reduce pain and to minimize the risk of further damage due to movement of broken bones.

Splints

See 'Splinting', p. 98 and 'Applying a splint', p. 99.

Spinal head hold

This is an instant temporary 'splint' for the victim's neck when a spinal injury is suspected. Hold the victim's head with both your forearms with your thumbs 'locked' over their collar bones, keeping the head, neck and spine completely still and in line. This spinal head hold is maintained until spinal injury is excluded (see 'Is this a serious spinal injury or can the victim move?', p. 86), or the head hold is replaced by suitable padding and bandaging on a stretcher (Fig 11.1).

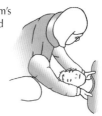

Fig 2.2 Spinal head hold

Ways to move a victim

Practise these techniques before you need to use them.

Spinal roll and spinal lift

This is the safest way to turn, or lift, a victim with a suspected spinal or head injury into the safe airway position (Fig 2.1) or onto a stretcher. The 'leader' applies a spinal head hold (Fig 2.2) and instructs the team of assistants on the procedure to follow, checking that each one has understood and is ready. On the leader's command, a slow coordinated roll or lift is carried out keeping the head, neck, shoulders, spine and hips in a straight line, avoiding bending or twisting of the victim's body.

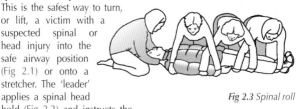

Fig 2.3 Spinal roll

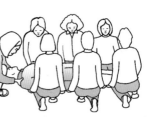

Fig 2.4 Spinal lift

One-person drag and quick roll

These techniques are used to drag an injured victim to safety or roll them into the safe airway position, when you are on your own. When doing the drag, if the victim is unconscious/semiconscious, tie their wrists together and loop them over your head around your neck.

See also Chapter 10, 'Evacuation'.

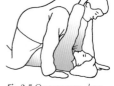

Fig 2.5 One-person drag

Fig 2.6 Quick roll

3. MEDICATIONS – WHAT YOU NEED TO KNOW

Each medication has only one *generic name*, usually found in small print somewhere on the original packaging, but may have many *trade names*. For example, 'ibuprofen' is the generic name of a medication which has many trade names such as Brufen™, Nurofen™, Fenbid™, Ibux™ etc. Use generic names as much as possible.

Medications often come in different strengths and release methods (eg slow/fast release). Always check the strength of your medication against those in this book and adjust your dose accordingly.

Medications are sometimes combined (eg Panadeine™ which is paracetamol and codeine in one tablet); try and avoid putting these in your first aid kit and be aware of this if you do.

Appendix 1 provides a Chart of Medications that covers most of the medications mentioned in the text, providing brief information on:

- the problems for which the medication is used
- the dosage (unless a * refers you to the text)
- some of the medication's side effects
- directions on how and when to take it.

Appendix 2 provides the above information for antibiotics.

Prescription-only medications

Some of the medications mentioned in this book are prescription-only. Use them only if:

- you are in a remote area and medical help is not available, *AND*
- a doctor has prescribed them with a written protocol, trained you directly to give the medication or advises you (via phone, radio, message) to give it, *AND*
- you have written informed consent from the victim (ie they understand you are not a doctor and the reason/risks involved), *AND*
- you have carried out a secondary survey, arrived at a diagnosis and the victim's condition is such that not giving the medication carries a substantial risk, *AND*
- you have checked the victim is not allergic to the medication and checked what other medications they may be taking for possible interreactions, *AND*
- you keep a careful written record of all the above.

Before departure ask your doctor/pharmacist about dangers, side effects and interactions with other medications, and check for antibiotic resistance. Always read the information on the medication's packaging and the leaflet inside. See 'Travelling with controlled drugs/medications', p. 12.

For more on first aid kits see Appendix 9; see also Appendix 10 – 'Travel Medicine and General Information' and Chapter 4 on pain management.

Ways to administer medications

- **By mouth** (oral): swallowing is the usual and simplest way to administer a medication. However, do not give medications (or liquids) by mouth to a victim who is unconscious/semiconscious. Injuries to the face/mouth may prevent use of the oral route.
- **Sublingual** (under the tongue) or buccal (inside the cheeks): some medications (eg fentanyl lozenges, Buccastem™) are absorbed through the mucosa (skin) of the mouth.
- **Inhaled** (eg asthma spray, methoxyflurane)
- **Enema**: this simple and potentially lifesaving procedure can be used to give medications, or rehydration liquids, via the victim's anus (ie up their bottom) into the victim's rectum, from where they are absorbed.
  ‣ The victim is positioned face down or on their side.
  ‣ Attach a suitable container or funnel to an 'enema tube' (a hydration pack with a flexible tube is a simple substitute) and fill it with the appropriate liquid.
  ‣ Lubricate the enema tube (with K-Y jelly, Vaseline™ or water) and gently insert it through the anal ring of muscles, no deeper than 3cm or half a finger length (measure and mark this length on the tube before insertion). By raising the funnel, the solution can be run into the victim's lower bowel (at a rate of no more than 200mls/hour, or a bit less than one cup/hour).
  ‣ Withdraw the tube, wash thoroughly, disinfect and dry ready for re-use.
  ‣ It is also possible to give small quantities of liquid containing a medication using a 2ml syringe (no needle, cut off the spike of the syringe), inserting the lubricated barrel gently into the anus.
- **Suppositories** (doses of medication in a waxy bullet shape): these are an effective way to administer medications through the anus into the rectum, and are particularly useful when vomiting, unconsciousness or injury prevents the oral route. They are best administered after a bowel movement, or at least an hour before.

▸ Position the victim on their side, knees drawn up.
▸ Wear gloves (or scrape fingernail in a bar of soap first if no gloves are available).
▸ Lubricate the suppository (K-Y jelly, vaseline or water) and push it up well past the anal muscle (half a finger length).

Note: enemas and suppositories are invasive and embarrassing procedures: obtain informed written consent before administration.

- **Nasogastric tubes** can be used for unconscious or semiconscious victims. Training is required.
- **Injections** can be intramuscular (IM), intravenous (IV) or subcutaneous (SC). Training is required.
- **Intravenous infusion**: training is required.
- **Skin application**: gels, ointments, creams and lotions. Some medications come as an adhesive skin patch (eg fentanyl).

Side effects and allergic reactions

A side effect is an unwanted effect or an allergic reaction caused by a medication. Before giving a medication:

- ask the victim whether they have any allergies, particularly to that medication
- ask them whether they are taking any other medication or recreational drugs: when two or more different medications are given together, they may interact (eg some strong painkillers plus antihistamines increase drowsiness)
- check the special risks of medications at altitude (see below).

Allergies to medications may range from mild (rash) to severe (see 'Anaphylactic shock', p. 67). As a general rule, if an allergic reaction develops, stop the medication and try an alternative. However, if the allergy to a medication is mild and the illness severe, and you have no alternative, you may still consider continuing to give it.

Common allergies to medications include:

- Penicillin allergy: avoid penicillin antibiotics eg amoxicillin, co-amoxiclav, flucloxacillin. A mild reaction is a rash, a severe reaction causes anaphylaxis. 10% of people with penicillin allergy react to the alternative cefalexin.
- Sulfa allergy: avoid co-trimoxazole antibiotics, use any of the other antibiotics recommended instead. Avoid silver sulfadiazine burn cream.

Acetazolamide (Diamox™) may (rarely) cause a sulfa allergic reaction: avoid in severe sulpha allergy.

- Aspirin and NSAID allergy: can provoke asthma, hives and generalized swelling.

Other first aid supplies that may cause an allergy include iodine, adhesive tape and latex examination gloves.

Special considerations

Children

There is *no information on medication doses for children in this book*. Parents need to obtain this information from their doctor or pharmacist. Children under 12 years old should NOT be given aspirin, ciprofloxacin, norfloxacin, tetracycline or doxycycline. Children under 9 years old should NOT be given Imodium™ or Lomotil™.

Pregnancy

Antibiotics may reduce the efficiency of oral contraceptives ('the pill'), so women taking the pill and an antibiotic should take other precautions until their next period.

Pregnant women should avoid malarial and Zika areas, and unnecessary medications. The antibiotics amoxicillin, erythromycin and cefalexin are relatively safe to use in pregnancy but avoid ciprofloxacin, co-trimoxazole, doxycycline, tetracycline, tinidazole, metronidazole, most antimalarial medications, acetazolamide (Diamox™) and iodine (for disinfecting water).

At altitude

In general

- At altitude (above 2500m) any medication that depresses respiration may make altitude illness more likely or worse, especially at night. Examples are the opiates (codeine etc), some sleeping medications and older antihistamines such as chlorphenamine (Piriton™). If you have to use any of these medications, consider giving acetazolamide (Diamox™) 125mg two hours before bedtime to stimulate breathing (see 'Drugs used for altitude illness' p. 171).
- Altitude seems to increase the side effects of some antimalarial medications, causing nausea and, occasionally, psychotic episodes (mefloquine).

- Oral contraceptives ('the pill') slightly increase the blood's tendency to clot, so avoid for longer stays above 5000m.

Acetazolamide (Diamox™)

Acetazolamide increases the respiratory rate at altitude and speeds up the acclimatization process, reducing the likelihood of AMS. It is especially useful for slow acclimatizers. However, taking acetazolamide does *not* guarantee that altitude illness will not develop. Acetazolamide does *not* mask the onset of AMS, HACE or HAPE. Acetazolamide appears to reduce maximum physical performance somewhat, especially in older people (50+), so keep the dose to an effective minimum. While its routine preventative use for all trekkers on all treks is *not* recommended, it is recommended for:

- those who have a past history of altitude illness
- slow acclimatizers (ie those suffering symptoms despite having followed a reasonable ascent profile)
- anyone suffering from periodic breathing (see 'Periodic breathing', p. 166)
- flying or driving rapidly to altitudes above 3000m (such as Lhasa 3660m, Leh 3500m, Cuzco 3470m or La Paz 3880m), especially when expecting to exercise hard on arrival (eg rescue or military teams).

Dosage: the preventative dose of acetazolamide varies from 125mg 12-hourly to 250mg 8-hourly; start with the lower dose and increase if symptoms persist. A dose takes 12 hours to become fully effective. For periodic breathing, one dose two hours before sleeping is often sufficient. Climbers on summit days should consider the balance between its positive and negative effects. If flying to altitude, start 24 hours before the flight and continue till descending from the trip highpoint or, cautiously, three days after arrival at altitude. Rapid response SAR and military teams should consider taking 250mg at least 12-hourly.

Allergy and side effects

Avoid acetazolamide if there is a history of a severe allergic reaction to sulfa-containing medications (mainly the sulphonamide-type antibiotics such as co-trimoxazole, Septrin™, Bactrim™). If the sulfa allergy is mild, test doses of acetazolamide (125mg 12-hourly for 2 days) may be tried well before departure (but do not attempt this if the sulfa allergy is severe!). It appears that most people with mild sulfa allergy can take acetazolamide without risk.

Common side effects of acetazolamide include the following:
- paraesthesia (tingling) in lips, fingers, toes or other body parts and a metallic taste when drinking carbonated drinks
- photosensitivity (tendency to sunburn more easily) so use hats, gloves, sunscreen
- extra urine output – this effect is mild (**Note:** people do pee more as part of the normal acclimatization process)
- rarer side effects include: flushing, headache, dizziness, nausea, diarrhoea, tiredness.

Note: the lower the dose, the milder the side effects which slowly disappear on stopping the medication. Using slow release acetazolamide reduces side effects.

4. PAIN MANAGEMENT

Finding yourself without the means to relieve someone's pain is wilderness medicine nightmare. Apart from being unpleasant, pain causes distress and can prevent you from carrying out important procedures/treatments. It is important to assess the severity of pain regularly in order to give the appropriate painkiller.

The signs of severe pain include inability to focus on anything other than the pain, fast heart rate, distressed facial expression and reluctance to move the painful part. Ask the victim to rate their pain on a scale of 1 to 10 (1 being no pain, 10 being the worst pain imaginable by the victim). Using changes in the above signs and scale over time will help judge deterioration or improvement.

Situations needing pain relief
- Acute trauma: wounds, burns, broken bones, dislocations, sprains
- Acute organ pain: gall, kidney and bladder stones/infection, heart attack, infections (meningitis, abscess, dengue fever), toothache, earache
- Carrying out a procedure: cleaning, removing dead or damaged tissue (debriding) and dressing wounds, removing splinters, amputating a mangled finger or toe, replacing dislocations, splinting broken bones, removing a superficial foreign object from an eye, dental work
- Milder aches and pains: simple headache, muscle aches, sore throat

Requirements for effective pain relief
- Right attitude: the positive effect of a calm, confident and reassuring attitude to pain relief cannot be overemphasized; without telling lies, reassure the victim that you will help them, and distract them by talking and/or holding their hand
- Right supportive technique: warmth, cooling, splinting fractures, compression, dressing, massage
- Right painkiller: chosen to suit the diagnosis after a careful secondary survey
- Right dose of painkiller: it is better to eliminate pain with adequate regular doses than to allow the pain to 'break through', requiring extra doses to regain control
- Right way to administer painkiller: choose the fastest and safest way, depending on your skill level. In order of simplicity, pain relief may be given by mouth, sublingual/buccal, inhaled, nasal spray, suppository

or injection (IM, IV, SC). Other ways are via the skin (gel or patch) or by enema

If the victim is in severe pain, is very stressed, has impaired swallowing, is vomiting regularly or has facial/mouth injuries, giving pain relief by mouth may be impossible, too slow or inefficient: use an alternative way.

Painkillers (analgesics)

General considerations

- There are many painkillers available, but only a few (such as paracetamol, ibuprofen, naproxen and codeine) are suitable for use by a non-medical person in a remote setting. However, with suitable training methoxyflurane (Penthrox™) and tramadol would be safe additions.
- Paracetamol, ibuprofen (or naproxen) and codeine (or tramadol) taken alone, or in combination, will treat nearly all but the more severe pain. They are reasonably safe if you follow the instructions. When combining painkillers it is vital that you do NOT give two different NSAIDs together: see 'Non-steroidal anti-inflammatory drugs (NSAIDS)' below.
- The strongest painkillers are controlled, prescription-only drugs and need special training for their use. In a wilderness setting, with potential for severe traumatic injury with pain, non medics with suitable training should be able to use fentanyl lozenges and methoxyflurane.
- Fast acting painkillers need to be eventually replaced by longer acting ones for persistent severe pain.
- All doses given in this book refer to adults only. Always check for allergy to painkillers.

Painkillers recommended

Paracetamol (acetaminophen, Panadol™, Tylenol™)
- The dose is 1000mg (two tabs) 4 to 6-hourly, to a maximum of 8 tabs in 24 hours.
- If this is not controlling the pain, add ibuprofen or codeine for a more powerful effect.

Side effects and cautions
- Do NOT give more than 16 tabs in 24 hours as it can cause liver damage.
- It can cause a rash.

Ibuprofen

- The dose is 200–400mg 6 to 8-hourly (for severe pain, the first two doses can be 800mg then reduced to the usual amount).
- The maximum dose in 24 hours is 2400mg (do not give this maximum dose for more than a few days).

If ibuprofen alone is not controlling the pain, add paracetamol or codeine for a more powerful effect (but do NOT give ibuprofen with aspirin or any of the other NSAIDs).

Note: some countries sell ibuprofen as 600mg tablets. ALWAYS check the strength of your medication against the dose recommended in this book. Naproxen and diclofenac are stronger then ibuprofen.

NON-STEROIDAL ANTI-INFLAMMATORY DRUGS (NSAIDS)

This includes ibuprofen (Brufen™, Nurofen™, Fenbid™, Ibux™), aspirin, diclofenac (Voltarol™), naproxen (Naprosyn™, Mobic™, Celebrex™), parecoxib (Dynastat™) etc.

NSAID painkillers reduce inflammation (with or without infection) and are used for muscle or bone pain (eg sprains, strains, bruising, trekker's knee, broken bones, dislocations), gall bladder, kidney, menstrual pain, headache (including AMS headache), migraine, sore throat, toothache. The painkilling effect of an NSAID starts right away and builds up over several doses. The full anti-inflammatory effect comes on more slowly – over a week or so. Larger doses are needed for inflammation.

Side effects and cautions of NSAIDs

- They are best given with food to a well-hydrated victim.

- They can make asthma worse or bring on an attack. Avoid NSAIDs in asthmatics unless they have taken them before. Be alert for wheezing/shortness of breath.

- Do not give to pregnant women or anyone with heart or kidney disease.

- For people over 65 years, halve the dose and give for the shortest possible time (or use paracetamol).

- NSAIDs can cause bleeding in the stomach so avoid if there is a history of (or active) peptic ulcers, heartburn or severe indigestion. Stop it if indigestion occurs.

43

- NSAIDs can cause nausea, rashes, fluid retention and dizziness.
- Use NSAIDs sparingly at very high altitude, and for the shortest possible time.

Note: different NSAIDs should never be given together.

Codeine phosphate

Codeine is used for mild to moderate pain. It can take the edge off severe pain, once the cause has been dealt with (eg a well-splinted fracture, or a cooled and covered burn).

- The adult dose of codeine phosphate is 15–60mg 4 to 8-hourly (maximum dose is 240mg in 24 hours).
- Start with a low dose, increasing it until effective.
- If codeine alone is not controlling the pain, add ibuprofen OR paracetamol for a more powerful effect.

Note: some paracetamol preparations are already mixed with codeine, do NOT add codeine to such mixtures.

THE OPIATES

Opiates are derived from opium poppies or are similar synthetics. They are controlled drugs (except tramadol and codeine in some countries) and appropriate custom forms must be carried (see 'Travelling with controlled drugs/medications' p. 12). They include codeine, morphine, heroin and the synthetic opiates tramadol, oxycontin and fentanyl. Opiates are not addictive after short-term use for pain. The stronger opiates are used for severe pain (burns, fractures, major trauma etc) and severe organ pain (heart attack, kidney and gall bladder stones etc).

Apart from codeine, specific and detailed training is needed before using opiates.

Opiate side effects and cautions

Do not give during an asthma attack, or for head injury or altitude illness (if they must be used at high altitude, see 'At altitude' p. 38).

- Depression of breathing occurs with higher doses. If carrying powerful opiates, also carry the overdose antidote Narcan™.
- Drowsiness is common as well as constipation (be ready with laxatives).
- Only consider codeine for abdominal pain if constipation has been excluded as the cause, and the victim is having normal bowel movements.
- Nausea or vomiting, dizziness, dry mouth, blurred vision, anxiety, confusion or agitation may occur.
- Do not give opiates with alcohol, sedatives, sleeping pills, sedating antihistamines or prochlorperazine (Stemetil™), as the combination depresses breathing even more.

Methoxyflurane (Penthrox™)
This is an inhaled painkiller. It is simple to use, after appropriate training, and an effective means of providing short-term pain relief in acute trauma, burns or painful procedures such as setting bones, relocating dislocated joints. It is used extensively by paramedics, ski patrollers, armed forces and industry first aiders in many countries (see Appendix 10).

Side effects and cautions
- It may cause nausea and dizziness. The first few breaths may feel harsh with a strong fruity smell.
- It does not depress breathing, even at altitude.
- It causes kidney damage if overused: do NOT exceed two 3ml ampoules in one day or a total of five 3ml ampoules in one week.
- Do NOT use methoxyflurane with tetracycline antibiotics.

Brief instructions: with the inhaler tilted up at 15° (mouthpiece down), pour the 3ml of liquid methoxyflurane into the cotton wool. Give (or toss, if the victim is inaccessible) to the victim. The vapour is inhaled intermittently, the victim judging his or her own need for pain relief. For extra strength, the victim may cover the small diluter hole. One ampoule lasts approximately 25 minutes of continuous use, and up to four hours of intermittent use.

Other painkillers

Those specifically trained should consider carrying:

- Morphine for injection and fentanyl lozenges
- Parecoxib (Dynastat™), an injectable NSAID, which gives excellent pain relief without the controlled drug customs restriction
- Lidocaine injection is used for local anaesthesia, regional nerve block or IV regional anaesthesia
- Ketamine IM/IV is used for pain relief and as a general anaesthetic, and is used for painful procedures such as minor surgery, treating fractures and dislocations: it appears not to affect respiration up to at least 5000m.

Other medications and techniques for pain relief

Other medications

There are several medications that can assist or replace painkillers, such as:

- simple antacids or ranitidine for indigestion pain, especially heartburn
- anaesthetic eye drops for eye pain due to foreign body or scratched cornea, eg lidocaine or tetracaine (Amethocaine™)
- Strepsil™ lozenges or aspirin gargles for sore throat.

Cooling treatment

Cold can be applied directly to the body using cold packs, bagged snow or ice (covered in cloth), or cold water compresses. It has several uses:

- reducing swelling and pain of sprains and strains
- giving short-lived (1 minute or so) pain relief, or anaesthetizing skin
- reducing the pain of certain jellyfish stings and some spider, scorpion and centipede bites.

Note: beware of frostbite and hypothermia when using these cooling techniques.

Heat application

Direct application of heat by means of packs or hot water baths, showers or compresses is useful for:

- relieving painful muscle spasm
- relieving the severe pain caused by some venomous fish, jellyfish, spiders etc. See p.129 and Appendix 7.

PART 2: ACCIDENT AND ILLNESS PROTOCOL

5. ACCIDENT AND ILLNESS PROTOCOL IN A WILDERNESS SETTING

It is natural to feel anxious and overwhelmed when suddenly confronted with an accident or severe illness. The protocol outlined here is for a remote wilderness setting.

In a major incident where there are helpers, you, as the lead first responder, should be observing, assessing, delegating and instructing, only becoming involved with a specific problem when unavoidable.

ACCIDENT AND ILLNESS PROTOCOL

1. Take control
2. Primary survey – dealing with life-threatening emergencies (Chapter 6) and Primary survey for specific situations (Chapter 7)
3. Shock prevention and stabilization (Chapter 8)
4. Secondary survey – working out what the problem is (Chapter 9)
5. Plan of action
6. Treatment
7. Evacuation (Chapter 10)

1. Take control

Stop and get a grip on yourself, calming down with a few deep breaths while resisting the urge to rush in. *Observe* the situation:

- **Danger:** Are you, the victim and the rest of the group safe from further injury, such as falls, rock falls, avalanche, water dangers, electrical appliances, power cables and road traffic? If not, act to rectify the situation immediately, calling for nearby help and delegating as much as possible.
- **Mechanism of injury (MOI):** Assess how the injury occurred and the forces involved. Could there be a neck or spinal injury? If not sure, assume there is. If there is more than one victim, assess who needs help first (triage).

Approach the victim:

- Do this from below or the side to avoid dislodging rocks, snow etc onto them, and so they can see you without turning their head (to avoid worsening a possible neck injury).
- Wear protective gloves.
- Ask the victim, 'Can I help you?' The response, or lack of it, tells you about the airway and level of consciousness. It also provides **consent**. If they say 'no', go no further. Assume consent if the victim is unconscious, semiconscious, drunk, or 'not of sound mind' ie suffering mental problems. If consent is given (or assumed), place your hand gently on their head to stabilize the neck, ask them to stay still and proceed.

MECHANISM OF INJURY (MOI)

The way an accident happened will help to work out the type and severity of injuries sustained. It is especially important in spinal and head injuries (Chapter 11). The MOI is also useful when considering broken bones, dislocations, sprains and strains (Chapter 13) and wounds (Chapter 14). Give some thought to the trajectory and weight of any striking object, to the position of the victim's body and how it arrived in the position you found it, and which vital organs lie under the injured area. Always consider the MOI when making a diagnosis (Chapter 9).

While there is plenty to consider in this first step, it should be accomplished quickly, in seconds rather than minutes, as the next step, the primary survey, is lifesaving and must be implemented as soon as possible.

2. Primary survey – dealing with life-threatening emergencies (Chapters 6 and 7)

Stop any deadly (life-threatening) bleeding, assess and maintain the victim's airway and breathing, giving CPR/chest compressions if necessary. A traditional way to remember the steps of primary survey is 'DRSABCS' (see 'Basic life support (BLS)' p. 52).

PART 2: Accident and illness protocol

3. Shock prevention and stabilization (Chapter 8)

Reassure the victim and keep them calm. Protect from the environment (heat, cold, rain, wind etc) and give adequate pain relief (eg splint fractures, give painkillers).

4. Secondary survey – working out what the problem is (Chapter 9)

Now gather and record all the information you need to make a diagnosis: take a medical history (including the victim's previous medical history), carry out a physical examination, check the vital signs and reconsider the MOI.

5. Plan of action

Once the victim is safe, the life-threatening emergencies have been dealt with, shock prevention is in place and ongoing, all relevant information has been gathered and a diagnosis made (if you have one!), decide on your plan of action. Consult your companions, read as much as you can about the problem and seek medical advice by phone, radio, email or messenger. Get the victim's consent, and their opinion on the plan as appropriate. Write down your plan of action, which might include some or all of the following:

- all treatments and care you have already given and intend to give (wound care, dressings, splinting, medications, liquids, nursing, posture, toilet needs, feeding etc)
- how you intend to continue shock prevention
- how often and when you will repeat the vital signs and secondary survey
- an inventory of your resources (equipment and skills of your group and what's locally available)
- how medical help or advice will be sought
- how evacuation will be organized and rescue request written
- how you will deal with all the possible things that could go wrong
- how you will deal with the needs of the rest of your group: briefings, food, shelter, evacuate/continue, keeping group morale positively directed by assigning jobs, debrief.

Review your plan of action regularly, especially when conditions change. And, for legal reasons, remember the saying 'if it wasn't written down (preferably as soon as possible), it wasn't done'.

6. Treatment

Now it's time to start your non-emergency treatments.

   If the treatment is ongoing, move the victim into the best possible space (eg mess tent on an expedition, good room in a lodge) as soon as it is safe to do so. Someone may need to stay with the victim during the night: arrange a roster. Record all treatments, vital signs, times, doses etc.

7. Evacuation (Chapter 10)

If the victim's condition is serious, deteriorating, or you or the victim cannot cope with the situation, evacuation will be necessary.

6. PRIMARY SURVEY – DEALING WITH LIFE-THREATENING EMERGENCIES

Providing basic life support (BLS) can save a life. In a wilderness situation CPR works well for drowning (submersion), avalanche victims, lightning strike, electrocution or choking.

What follows is a reminder to the trained rescuer, and a guide to the untrained (have someone read the steps of BLS below).

DEFINITIONS

- **Basic life support** (BLS): techniques for controlling deadly bleeding, and resuscitating a person who is not breathing or whose heart has stopped beating
- **Rescue breathing** (also called mouth-to-mouth or expired air resuscitation – EAR): using the rescuer's breath to ventilate the victim's lungs (this is effective without previous training)
- **Chest compressions:** squeezing the heart to provide blood circulation when the heart has stopped (this is effective without previous training)
- **Cardiopulmonary resuscitation** (CPR): a combination of rescue breathing and chest compressions (best learned before you need to use it)

BASIC LIFE SUPPORT (BLS)

A way to remember everything is 'DRSABCS'.

D = Deadly bleeding: check for and treat any life-threatening bleeding.

R = Response: check whether the victim is conscious, semiconscious or unconscious.

S = Send for help (if help is nearby).

A = Airway: open, clear and maintain a safe, effective airway into the lungs.

B = Breathing: check whether they are breathing.

C = Circulation: start chest compressions and rescue breathing (CPR) as necessary.

S = Specific situations: situations that require specific responses – see Chapter 7.

D = Deadly bleeding

Check for and treat any life-threatening bleeding: sweep your hands (using protective gloves) gently but thoroughly over and under the whole of the victim's body. Check your gloves for blood after each area of the body is explored. Feel inside bulky clothing, as it can absorb large amounts of blood. If you find a source of life-threatening bleeding, control it (p. 58) before continuing your search.

R = Response

Determine whether the victim is conscious, semiconscious or unconscious by checking their response to '*touch and talk*': gently squeeze the victim's (uninjured) shoulder, while keeping a hand on their forehead to prevent neck movement, and ask loudly, 'Can I help you?'

- A clear spoken reply means they are *conscious* and breathing normally.
- If the response is vague, unclear or absent they are *semiconscious* or *unconscious*.

IF THE VICTIM IS CONSCIOUS WITH NORMAL BREATHING, continue with shock prevention and stabilization (Chapter 8).

IF THE VICTIM IS SEMICONSCIOUS OR UNCONSCIOUS, continue with the following steps.

S = Send for help

If help is nearby.

A = Airway

- **Turn** the victim on their back (if not possible, do the best you can in position found).
- **Clear** their mouth of any blockage (blood, vomit etc).
- **Open** the victim's airway.

OPENING (AND MAINTAINING) THE VICTIM'S AIRWAY

- Gently *tilt* the victim's head back.
- *Grip* under the point of their chin with your fingers and lift it away from their throat/neck (or use jaw thrust).
- *Open* their mouth.

Note: no head tilt if a spinal injury is suspected, or for infants, unless needed to open the airway (in which case use the minimum tilt needed). This may be done with the victim in any other position (eg safe airway position).

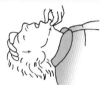

Fig 6.1 Opening the victim's airway

B = Breathing

Spend up to 10 seconds checking whether or not the victim is now breathing normally.
- *Look* for movement of the chest and belly.
- *Listen* for breath sounds at the victim's mouth.
- *Feel* for air against your cheek (and for breathing movement with your hand lightly on their belly).

Note: in the first minutes after a person's heart has stopped beating (ie they have died), they may still have barely detectable breathing or be making infrequent, noisy gasps. Do not confuse this with normal breathing, as it is a sign that the heart has stopped. If you have any doubts about the victim's breathing, consider it to be abnormal.

IF THE SEMICONSCIOUS OR UNCONSCIOUS VICTIM IS BREATHING NORMALLY AND WITHOUT DIFFICULTY, roll them into the safe airway position (Fig 2.1) and keep checking that their breathing is continuing normally. Continue with shock prevention and stabilization (see Chapter 8).

C = Circulation

IF THE VICTIM IS NOT BREATHING OR NOT BREATHING NORMALLY, start CPR or chest compressions.

CPR: start with 30 chest compressions followed by 2 rescue breaths. Continue this at a ratio of 30:2. Do not stop CPR to check for breathing or for a pulse.

Chest compressions only: if you are unwilling or unable to give rescue breathing, give chest compressions only.

CHEST COMPRESSIONS

- Place the heel of your hand in the middle of the chest at the centre of the breastbone (sternum) with your other hand on top of it.

- Compress the chest 4–5cm (1½–2 inches) or one-third of chest depth. Keep your arms straight and the heel of your hand touching the chest at all time, without bouncing.

- The rate should be 100/min (a little slower than 2 compressions/ second).

- In CPR, there should be no pause between compressions and breaths.

- Do not stop to check for a pulse: if the victim's heart starts beating effectively again,

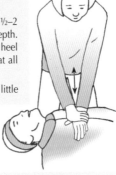

Fig 6.2 Chest compressions

there will be obvious positive changes of skin colour (white or blue will change to pink), or the victim will start moving, or their breathing will return.

RESCUE BREATHING

Fig 6.3 Rescue breathing

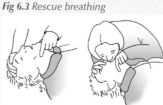

- Open the airway (see box above).
- Place your mouth over the victim's mouth and block their nose with your fingers.
- Blow in their mouth, enough to make their chest rise, sensing when their lungs are full.
- Wait until their chest has fallen before giving a second breath.

Note: if the chest doesn't rise, re-position the head and neck. Whether the breaths are effective or not, after two breaths continue with chest compressions.

When there are two first aiders

Take turns giving CPR; change roles every two minutes to make it most effective.

When to stop CPR or chest compressions?

It is acceptable to stop when:

- medical help arrives and takes over
- you are exhausted, or after 30 minutes (longer if a child is involved)
- the safety of you or your group is at risk
- a hypothermic victim has been re-warmed and there are still no signs of life.

IF THE VICTIM STARTS BREATHING NORMALLY, roll them into the safe airway position, making sure their airway is open. Continue to monitor their breathing.

S = Specific situations

See next chapter.

ASSISTED BREATHING

This is rescue breathing given BEFORE the victim stops breathing. In a wilderness setting, there are several critical situations where this can be lifesaving:

- breathing is slowing down and level of consciousness is falling
- colour of victim's skin or mucosa (inside lips, mouth, eyelid) is changing to white or blue
- victim is becoming exhausted
- severe altitude illness
- hypothermic victim (give gentle assisted breathing).

Giving assisted breathing

- If the victim is conscious, explain what you are going to do and get consent. Encourage them to relax: tell them, 'Let me breathe for you'.
- Give rescue breathing, preferably via a face mask or shield, but if necessary mouth-to-mouth. In hypothermia, mouth-to-mouth is preferable to mechanical ventilation (Ambu bag™ etc), as the expired air is warmed and that heat goes to exactly the right place.

PART 2: Accident and illness protocol

7. PRIMARY SURVEY FOR SPECIFIC SITUATIONS

Some situations require a modification or addition to the standard primary survey:

- suspected spinal injuries
- deadly (life-threatening) bleeding
- choking (blocked airway)
- road accident
- drowning (submersion)
- hypothermia
- avalanche victim
- primary survey for children
- loss of consciousness/semi-consciousness
- triage (more victims than first aiders).

Suspected spinal injuries

If a spinal injury is suspected:

- keep the victim in the position you find them and keep them as still as possible
- stop any movement of the head and neck by applying a spinal head hold (Fig 2.2), or by using your knees to gently hold their head still
- if you must move the victim (eg dangerous or inaccessible location, or to gain vital access), use spinal lifts or rolls (See Chapter 2)
- if opening the airway, use jaw thrust OR only tilt the head if needed and then only by the minimum necessary.

Spinal immobilization techniques must now be continued without interruption until a spinal injury has been excluded (see 'Is this a serious spinal injury or can the victim move?', p. 86 and also 'Pelvis' p. 107).

Deadly (life-threatening) bleeding

Controlling bleeding by direct pressure

This is an effective way to encourage blood vessels to contract and enable clot formation. Elevating the bleeding part may also help.

- Apply firm pressure directly on the bleeding area to stop it. The pressure may need to be very firm. Use (gloved) fingers or hand(s) directly or via a pad of dressing material (this may then be bandaged tightly in place). Check CSMS (see 'Checking CSMS', p. 74). Subsequent layers of dressing and bandage may be added on top.

- To assist control of the bleeding, keep the victim still, lie them down, immobilize the part.
- Once applied, do not release the pressure for at least 20 minutes by your watch (the first clot forms fastest due to a high concentration of clotting factors early on in the bleed, so do not give in to the temptation to 'take a peek' as fresh bleeding can wash away a half-formed clot).
- If bleeding restarts after 20 minutes of pressure, repeat the process. It can take up to two hours of repeated pressure to stop bleeding.

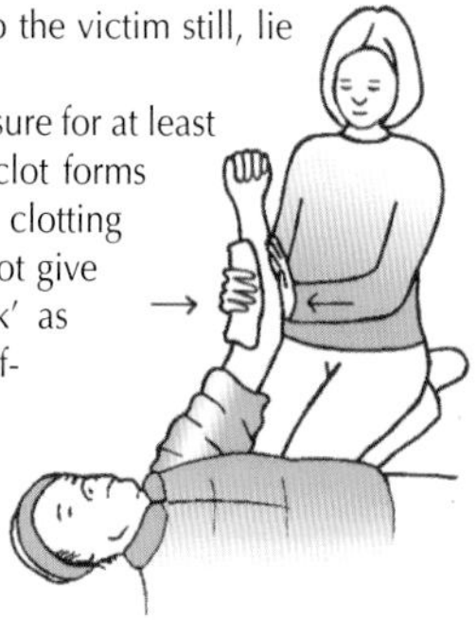

Fig 7.1 Controlling bleeding by direct pressure

Controlling life-threatening bleeding with a tourniquet

There are some situations when it is impossible to control bleeding from a limb using direct pressure. Usually this is due to traumatic amputation, massive wounds, multiple wounds, open fractures or penetrating wounds. When life-threatening bleeding from a limb continues, a tourniquet is essential. This is applied until direct pressure is effective or medical help is available. Only use a tourniquet if you and the victim understand the danger that this may be a choice between 'life or limb'.

A tourniquet is most efficient when applied to the upper arm or leg, less so on the lower arm or leg, where two bones prevent efficient arterial compression.

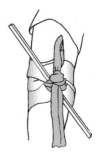

Fig 7.2 Controlling bleeding with a tourniquet

- Leaving the pressure dressing in place, position the tourniquet at least 10cm above the bleeding site, but not over a joint.
- Put something broad (5–10 cm wide) and strong (strap, scarf, bandage or triangular bandage) around the limb a couple of times and tie in a simple knot (half hitch). Place a lever (eg a stick) across the knot and tie a couple of simple knots over it. Now rotate the lever to tighten the tourniquet, compressing the artery until bleeding stops and no pulse can be

felt beyond the tourniquet. This can be very painful, so warn the victim and offer appropriate pain relief. Write down the time the tourniquet was applied and pass this information on to subsequent rescuers.

- If medical help is immediately available (within three hours) leave the tourniquet in place. The only person then allowed to remove the tourniquet is the doctor who takes over care for the victim.
- In a remote setting with no medical help: after 30 minutes apply direct pressure to the dressings over the bleeding point and release the tourniquet. Re-apply the tourniquet if life-threatening bleeding continues, and try releasing again after a further 30 minutes.

As a lifesaving last resort you might have to leave a tourniquet in place. This will result in the death of the limb and subsequent amputation. Consider this drastic action only if:
- medical help is unavailable
- bleeding continues despite direct pressure, and shock and death is likely
- you have explained to the victim, next-of-kin or friends that this will result in the subsequent amputation of the limb and they have given their consent.

Choking (blocked airway)
Choking is caused by inhaling a foreign object (eg food). The blockage of the airway may be mild or severe. A common choking scenario is a person drinking alcohol, eating and talking at the same time.

Symptoms and signs
- The victim may be clutching their neck or pointing (often frantically) at their neck or mouth.
- **Mild blockage:** the victim can speak, cough and breathe, but breathing is noisy and/or difficult.
- **Severe blockage:** this is a total obstruction. The victim:
  ‣ cannot breathe, or breathing is difficult, wheezing or noisy
  ‣ cannot speak, but may nod or shake head in response to questions
  ‣ cannot cough properly (attempts to cough are silent or ineffective)
  ‣ becomes unconscious.

Management
Immediate recognition that this is choking (and not a faint or heart attack) is vital. Ask the victim, 'Are you choking?'. A nod confirms your course of action:

Mild blockage

- Do NOT use back blows or abdominal thrusts, as they may make the blockage worse. Reassure them while encouraging them to lean forward (head below hips if they can manage it) and cough up the obstructing object. If this is not possible, evacuate for treatment.

Severe blockage

- If the victim is conscious but not breathing, give up to 5 sharp back blows (in the middle of the back, between the shoulder blades) while supporting the front of the victim's chest with the other hand and leaning them forward and down. Check for improvement.

- If this doesn't work, give 5 chest thrusts (these are similar to the chest compressions of CPR, with the heel of one hand in the middle of the chest, but the compressions are given at a slower rate and in a sharper manner).

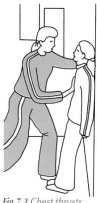

- If there is still no improvement, perform the Heimlich manoeuvre.
  - ▸ The victim may be sitting or standing.
  - ▸ Stand behind the victim. Encircle their waist with your arms, making a fist with one hand and place it slightly above the victim's navel and below their breastbone.
  - ▸ Grasp your fist with your other hand and quickly/forcefully pull in and up into the victim's upper abdomen (belly), letting the victim's upper body fall forward as you do so. This pushes air out of their lungs and will hopefully expel the obstructing object.

Fig 7.3 Chest thrusts

Note: chest thrusts and the Heimlich manoeuvre may cause internal damage.

- If the victim becomes unconscious place them onto their back, open their airway and try to see the obstructing object, hooking it out with your fingers, forceps or

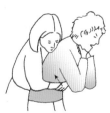

Fig 7.4 Abdominal thrusts (Heimlich manoeuvre)

tweezers. If this is not possible, start CPR as chest compressions can expel an obstruction.

- A trained rescuer may consider performing an emergency cricothyroidotomy.
- **For choking children**, use the same treatment as above but no abdominal thrusts if they are under one year old. Sit down, lay the baby face down along your thighs whilst supporting their head with your hands and give back blows as above.

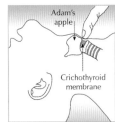

Note: after a successful treatment for choking, there may still be some foreign matter lodged in the victim's airway resulting in persistent cough, difficulty swallowing or a

Fig 7.5 Emergency cricothyroidotomy

persistent sensation of 'something being stuck in the throat'. In this case, evacuate for medical assessment.

Road accident

- Do not touch vehicles or victims within 10m of a fallen power line.
- Use hazard lights, road triangles or torches to warn traffic.
- Turn ignition off, apply parking brakes or chock the wheels.
- Manage unconscious breathing victims in the vehicle, opening their airway.
- Remove motorbike helmet to manage airway.
- If victim is unconscious and not breathing despite opening the airway, remove immediately from vehicle and commence CPR.

When removing the victim from the vehicle you will need to use the best spinal immobilization techniques you can manage (see Chapter 2 p. 33).

Drowning (submersion)

- Keep the victim horizontal and get them out of the water (only start rescue breathing while still in the water if you cannot get them out immediately).
- Place them on their back and start CPR (30:2).

See more on drowning p. 174.

Hypothermic victim

See 'Hypothermia' p. 132.

Avalanche victim

Rescuers must act swiftly but safely. With no other injuries, survival is good if extrication occurs within 15 minutes. See Appendix 4.

Primary survey for children

When doing a primary survey on a child, the force of breaths and compressions must be adjusted to the size of the child. The same steps of BLS must be followed, except:

- don't apply head tilt
- apply just enough force to compress the chest about one-third of its depth (using two fingers, one hand, or both hands as appropriate)
- for babies and small children, cover both their mouth and nose with your mouth.

Loss of consciousness/semi-consciousness

There are many non-traumatic causes of reduced levels of consciousness, such as anaphylaxis, hypoglycaemia in diabetics, heart attack, epileptic fits, heat and cold problems etc, but the commonest is a simple faint.

Fainting is a brief reversible loss of consciousness due to a fall in blood pressure and subsequent reduction in blood supply to the brain. Fainting can be caused by strong emotions (eg bad news, sight of blood, injections), standing still too long (especially in hot weather and after running), pain etc.

Correct treatment leads to rapid recovery, although the victim may feel weak or dizzy for some hours afterwards and may faint again.

Treatment

- Safe airway position and raise their legs slightly.
- In a hot climate check for heat injury (see Chapter 17).
- Carry out a secondary survey to exclude or identify other illnesses.

Triage

Triage means categorising multiple victims.

- Assess each victim as quickly as possible (a minute or so) and carry out these urgent simple lifesaving procedures:
  ‣ check for response, and place any unconscious or semiconscious victim in the safe airway position (Fig 2.1)
  ‣ clear and open the airway (Fig 6.1)

PART 2: Accident and illness protocol

‣ deal quickly with any obvious life-threatening bleeding (eg by tying something firmly over a bleeding point or by applying a tourniquet, Fig 7.2). The victim or bystanders can help with this.

Chest compressions and rescue breathing are NOT given at this point (exception: in **lightning strike** when apparently-dead victims are given CPR as a priority).

- Once all the victims have been assessed, quickly prioritize the victims needing further urgent treatment.
- Start shock prevention and stabilization (Chapter 8) using bystanders.
- Finally, consider giving CPR to the remaining unresponsive victims.

8. SHOCK PREVENTION AND STABILIZATION

Shock

Shock, in the medical sense, is a specific life-threatening physical condition caused by inadequate circulation of oxygenated blood to vital organs, leading to tissue damage. It is NOT an emotional or psychological state. There are many causes of shock and the aim is to recognize the potential for shock and prevent it as, once established, death from shock is certain.

Common causes of shock
- Bleeding: external or internal (especially from lacerated or torn organs, or from a broken pelvis/femur)
  - Estimating blood loss: if there is a lot of blood around the victim assume one litre of blood loss, then add another litre each for: a broken long bone (leg or arm); a broken pelvis; a chest injury; an abdominal injury.
  - Adults can tolerate a loss of up to one litre of blood; more than this can cause shock.
- Fluid loss: burns (plasma loss from the skin), severe diarrhoea, vomiting, severe sweating and dehydration
- Heart problems: heart attack, abnormal heart rhythm, electrocution, obstructive shock due to blocked blood flow into or out of the heart (tension pneumothorax, pulmonary embolus)
- Anaphylactic shock
- Spinal injury with severed spinal cord above the level of the mid-back
- Harness suspension trauma: this is due to pooling of blood in the abdomen and legs when a person hangs in a climbing harness: it comes on rapidly within 5 to 30 minutes
- Septic shock due to severe pneumonia, septicaemia

Symptoms and signs
- Dizziness, weakness, thirst, anxiety, restlessness, confusion, nausea, breathlessness, feeling cold
- Skin is (deathly) pale, white or grey (ashen) and is cool to touch. There is poor 'pink return' in the nails (see 'Checking CSMS', p. 74)
- Increasing pulse and respiratory rates
- Gums, tongue and lips are turning white or blue
- A falling level of consciousness
- Little or no urine output

MONITORING THE VICTIM'S PULSE AND RESPIRATORY RATES

This is the best guide to their condition and progress.

- Check the pulse rate at the wrist (or at the carotid or femoral arteries). If it is more than 100 beats per minute, there is something needing urgent attention such as blood loss, pain, fever, anxiety. Deal with whatever your secondary survey has found and continue to monitor the pulse. An easily felt pulse with a rate falling back toward normal means treatments are working. An increasing pulse rate, especially one getting hard to feel, is a bad sign.

  As an approximation, if a wrist pulse is easily felt the circulation is adequate. If wrist pulse cannot be felt the circulation is inadequate.

- Check the respiratory rate. A faster than normal rate (more than 25 breaths a minute) indicates shock (note that an increased respiratory rate occurs in shock even if the lungs are OK). An improving respiratory rate is a good sign.

- Deal with whatever your secondary survey has found and continue recording the respirations.

Note: young, fit adults with injuries can often maintain adequate blood pressure and look reasonably well, then collapse with shock very quickly!

Shock prevention and victim stabilization

What follows assumes that all immediately life-threatening emergencies have been dealt with and you are now stabilizing/improving the victim's condition before you start your secondary survey.

General treatment

- Keep the victim still and in the position found, or lie them down if they are staggering around. If lying down flat makes them more breathless (especially likely with heart problems or chest injury) try raising their head and shoulders or even sitting them up or turning them on their uninjured side (but see 'Chest injuries', p. 107). Ask them which position feels best. If unconscious, nurse in stable side position.

- Protect from the environment, providing shelter from wind, rain or heat (shade and ground insulation) and cold (insulation and warmth).

- Give ongoing reassurance to the victim by talking to them: explain what you are doing and why, but don't lie about their condition or 'talk over them', especially if discussing negative outcomes or serious injuries (even if they are semiconscious or unconscious).

Specific treatment

- Give oxygen (6 to 10L/min): this is very effective. Or give assisted breathing (see 'Assisted breathing', p. 57).
- Give effective pain relief as soon as possible. This means:
  ‣ splint broken bones, cool burns etc
  ‣ give adequate pain relief (see Chapter 4).
- Remove/cut off enough clothing to find major injuries while minimizing movement (the exception is a fractured pelvis, see 'Pelvis' p. 107).
- Maintain hydration as appropriate (Chapter 18).

GIVING LIQUIDS BY MOUTH?

Give small, frequent sips of liquid by mouth ONLY if rescue is delayed more than 6 hours AND:

- the victim is fully alert and swallowing normally
- the problem is due to (now controlled) bleeding, diarrhoea or burns
- there is NO internal bleeding
- surgery needing a general anaesthetic is NOT going to take place in the next 6 hours.

Note: it is best NOT to give fluids at all if internal bleeding is suspected.

Anaphylactic shock

This is caused by an allergic reaction to a medication (especially if injected), insect sting, food or inhaled substance. It comes on rapidly and is life-threatening owing to a severe drop in blood pressure and breathing difficulties caused by tissue swelling in the airways.

Symptoms and signs

- Itching of the mouth and skin
- Swelling of face, tongue, throat and body
- Difficulty breathing: this is serious, as are the next two signs
- Blueness of lips, tongue or face

- Abdominal pain, nausea, vomiting
- Shock

Treatment

- Use the victim's own self-injecting epinephrine device (EpiPen™, Anapen™, Jext™ etc).

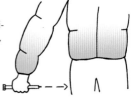

Fig 8.1 Using an EpiPen™

  ‣ Read the instructions.
  ‣ Form a fist around the device, with the black tip down.
  ‣ Pull off the grey activation cap with the other hand.
  ‣ Hold black tip near the victim's outer thigh, swing and jab firmly into outer thigh so that auto-injector is at a 90° angle to the skin surface.
  ‣ Hold it firmly in their thigh for 10 seconds to allow the epinephrine time to be absorbed. Remove and massage the area.
- If epinephrine (adrenaline) is not available, use phenylephrine or pseudoephedrine nasal spray or drops (8 to 10 sprays/drops in each nostril): repeat every 15 minutes until improvement occurs.
- For the medically trained: administer epinephrine (adrenaline) IM injection (0.3–0.5ml of 1:1000). Repeat every 15 minutes until improvement occurs. **Note:** NEVER give epinephrine (adrenaline) intravenously.
- For breathing difficulties, use a reliever asthma spray.
- Give oxygen (10 to 15L/min).
- Give prednisolone immediately, same dose as for asthma. If you have no prednisolone, use dexamethasone (dose as for HACE).
- Give an antihistamine.
- If the anaphylactic shock is due to a sting, remove the sting then apply a pressure immobilization bandage (PIB).
- If asthmatic and wheezy, give own reliever medication (salbutamol) via spacer.
- Evacuate, as any improvement may be followed by relapse (in which case start treatment again).

See also 'Toxic shock syndrome', p. 198.

9. SECONDARY SURVEY – WORKING OUT WHAT THE PROBLEM IS

A secondary survey is a systematic way to find the cause of the victim's problem (the **diagnosis**).

There are three parts to a secondary survey and the order in which they are carried out will depend on the situation:

- taking a full **medical history** – start with this if the victim has an illness
- carrying out a **physical examination** – start with this if they are injured
- checking the **vital signs** – start with this if they are unconscious or semiconscious.

Incident forms (downloadable from www.adventuremedicalconsulting.co.uk) are the best way to make sure nothing vital is missed or forgotten. Having gathered and recorded all this information, take your time to make a diagnosis.

You might be confident of a specific diagnosis, you might be unsure, or you might have no idea at all. If you don't have a firm diagnosis, keep an open mind: list the possibilities in order of probability and think of ways to check them out. Talk your ideas through with other team members (or even the victim), read up on and research the possibilities. Asking about changes in symptoms ('How are you now?' 'Has anything changed?' 'Have other symptoms appeared?') and repeating your examination and vital signs may eventually firm up your diagnosis. At the very least, time will tell you if the victim's condition is worsening, stable or improving.

Note: always check for hypothermia, exhaustion, dehydration, hypoglycaemia (and altitude illness if above 2500m), which are all common and share similar symptoms and signs. One or more of these easily treated conditions may be the diagnosis, or may be complicating a totally different problem.

DEFINITIONS

- **Symptoms:** what the victim feels. Symptoms are found by taking a medical history.
- **Signs:** what you can see, feel, smell, hear or measure, such as swelling, bruising, deformity, temperature, pulse/respiratory rate, urine colour and volume, level of consciousness. Signs are found by doing a physical examination and taking the vital signs.

Taking a medical history

Taking a medical history is the only way to arrive at the correct diagnosis when someone is ill. It is a skill that needs practise.

Ask the victim to tell you everything about their problem. If possible, talk to them privately in a quiet, well-lit, sheltered place. Speak clearly and ask simple questions, one at a time, and allow time for the answers. Below is a list of typical questions: use them as appropriate.

A traditional way to remember everything is 'SAMPLE'.

S = Symptoms

- Ask about and record the symptoms of their presenting condition: 'What is the problem?'
- 'When did it start? How did it start? How did it happen?'
- 'How are you feeling?'
- 'Describe the pain/symptom. Where is it? Does it move anywhere else? Is it coming and going? Is it getting better or worse? Have you taken anything for it? And if so, did this help or not?'
- 'What makes the pain/symptom better or worse?' (eg food, drink, position)
- 'How severe is the pain on a scale of 1 to 10 (1 being no pain at all, 10 being the worst pain you can imagine)?'
- 'Has this problem happened before? If so, what was it called and how was it treated?'
- 'Do you have any other problems?' (If so, repeat the questions above for each new problem/symptom.)
- At altitude, ask about AMS symptoms and complete the Lake Louise Score (see Appendix 6).
- Keep asking until all symptoms have been thoroughly checked out.
- Finally you might ask, 'What do YOU think the problem is?'

A = Allergies

'Are you allergic to anything (eg medications, food, stings, bites, pollen, adhesive tape)? What is your allergic reaction like? Do you think your present symptoms could be caused by your allergy?'

M = Medication/drugs

'Are you taking any medications? What for? What dose? Did a doctor prescribe them? Have you missed any medications you should be taking (especially antimalarial, diabetic and other regular medication)? Do you wear contact lenses? Have you been drinking alcohol or using any recreational drugs? Do you smoke?'

P = Past relevant medical history

'Do you have any medical conditions or illnesses (eg asthma, diabetes, epilepsy, high blood pressure, angina)? Have you been to the doctor in the last 12 months? If so, what for? Have you had any illnesses, injuries or operations in the past? When was your last tetanus shot?'.

L = Last 'ins and outs'

Ask the victim (as appropriate) about frequency, quantity and consistency over the last 24 hours, of the following:

- **Liquid intake:** 'How much have you drunk in the last 24 hours, including tea, coffee, soups etc? Is this normal for you?'
- **Urination:** 'Approximately how many times have you peed in the last 24 hours? What was the colour, amount and smell of your last pee?' (A healthy person will produce a minimum of one litre of clear or pale yellow and odourless urine every 24 hours.)
- **Food intake:** 'How much have you eaten in the last 24 hours? Is this normal for you?'
- **Bowel motions:** 'How many have you had in the last 24 hours? Is this normal for you?' Ask about volume, consistency (eg watery, porridge-like, 'normal'). 'Is there any blood or mucus? Are the motions black and tar-like? Is it explosive? Any pain during or after bowel motion?'
- **Vomit:** 'How many times/amount in the last 24 hours? Was it 'projectile', smelling like faeces, bloody?'
- **Menstruation:** If relevant, ask women about their last period, whether it was normal/missed (pregnancy?); ask if they are currently using tampons (toxic shock syndrome). 'Are you using contraception ('the pill', hormone injection, coil etc)?'

E = Events leading up to the injury or illness

How did it start? How did it happen? (See 'Mechanism of injury (MOI)', p. 49).

Carrying out a physical examination

A full physical examination consists of a complete and careful look and feel of the whole body (head to toe). A simple way to remember the basics is 'DOTS': Deformity, Open wounds, Tenderness, Swelling.

PART 2: Accident and illness protocol

The way you do a physical examination is decided by the victim's injury/ illness, and how much you can move them (eg spinal injuries, broken bones, drowning, hypothermia).

Take your time. Depending on circumstances (eg intimate examinations of the opposite sex), you may need a witness (eg victim's friend) present at all times (the witness doesn't need to hear all that is said, but they need to see all that is done).

If there has been an injury, special attention must be directed to the injured area. But also examine the rest of the body, as the pain of one injury may mask other less painful but possibly serious injuries.

- Take a general look at the victim: do they look well, unwell or seriously ill? Do they feel cold, feverish or clammy? Is their skin colour normal? Check wrists, neck, pockets and bags for medic-alert tag/medications/ID.
- Remove as much clothing and jewellery as needed for your examination, appropriate to the injury/illness and the situation/weather conditions.
- Systematically look, feel, smell and listen for anything abnormal. Specifically look for bleeding (control it), wounds, burns and broken bones (temporarily covering/splinting them before continuing), swelling, bruising, bites and stings, tenderness, discoloration rashes and the odours of alcohol and ketoacidosis (smells of almonds: see 'Hyperglycaemia', p. 208). Feel with the pads of your fingers and ask, 'Does it hurt?' Start with gentle pressure, finishing with a firm squeeze. Watch the victim's face for grimacing, screwing up eyes or groaning, or the withdrawing of an injured arm or leg, all signs of tenderness/pain (this is especially useful if the victim is semiconscious/unconscious). In order, examine the following:

  ‣ **Head and neck:** check around the head, face, neck and collarbones. Look behind the ears (for bruising), check for clear fluid from ears or nose (a sign of head injury with open fracture).

  ‣ **Chest:** check the front, sides and back of the chest. Ask the victim to take a deep breath: if this is painless, ask them to cough (pain at either of these steps is a sign of possible spinal, internal, chest or abdominal injury). If the cough was not painful, gently, then more firmly, compress the ribs by squeezing the rib cage from side to side and from front to back (pain is a sign of possible bruised or broken ribs, sternum or spinal injury).

  ‣ **Back and spine:** if you can reach the spine without moving the victim, press gently along it, from the top of their neck to the crack of their buttocks. Stop if there is any marked tenderness or pain at any point in this examination and assume there is a possible spinal injury (see Chapter 11).

▸ **Belly (abdomen):** gently, then more firmly, press on the abdomen with the flat of your hand at all four corners and the centre, noting any tenderness, rigidity or swelling. Ask them to breathe in deeply, then push out their belly, then cough. Stop if there is any tenderness or pain at any point in this examination and assume there is a possible abdominal, pelvic or spinal injury or serious abdominal problem.

▸ **Pelvis:** if there is no pelvic pain and no suspicion of a pelvic injury, place a hand on each pelvic crest (hipbone) and gently press them backwards, then towards each other. Then press on the pubic bone. Stop if any of this causes pain, as pelvic fractures bleed easily (splint immediately).

▸ **Arms and legs:** systematically feel the limbs all over. By comparing the injured with the uninjured limb, any colour changes or swelling/ deformity are much easier to detect (try closing your eyes and, with both your hands, gently examine the same position on both limbs at the same time). This will reveal any bone, joint or muscle injury. Check for changes to CSMS (see below). Once all major injuries have been excluded or stabilized, check their wrist, ankle, elbow, knee, shoulder and hip joints for tenderness and pain through a full range of active (the victim moves the joint themselves) and passive (you move their joint) movements.

■ If the victim lost consciousness: for how long? Do they have memory loss from before, during or after the injury?

■ Check for signs of hypothermia and dehydration.

■ At high altitude, check for altitude illness (see Chapter 22).

Write down (and/or draw diagrams) of all your findings. Consider taking photographs of any obvious injuries, especially frostbite at various stages (explain to the victim their value for advice by email and for follow-up treatment). Repeat your examination once the pain of major injuries has been controlled. Re-examine daily (or more frequently) if the victim is very ill, badly injured or getting worse.

CHECKING CSMS (CIRCULATION, SENSATION, MOVEMENT AND STRENGTH) IN LIMBS

Remember to compare with the uninjured limb.

- **C = *Circulation.*** When blood flow through a limb is reduced (by cold or shock) or cut off (due to compression/injury of blood vessels), the skin colour and temperature change. The limb becomes paler, white or bluish and feels cooler to touch compared to normal pinkness and warmth. Prolonged loss of circulation means the limb will die and infection will occur (eg from tourniquets, fractures, splints). Use the '**capillary circulation test**' to check the peripheral circulation in a limb: press on the victim's finger or toenail with your own fingernail for 5 seconds so the pink colour turns white; stop pressing and, if circulation is present and the victim is not too cold, the pink colour will rapidly return (within 2 seconds). If this 'pink return' does not occur, or takes longer than 5 seconds to fully return, it means that the circulation in the limb is inadequate.

- **S = *Sensation.*** Changed sensation in a limb suggests spinal or nerve damage (due to compression/injury) and/or loss of circulation. Ask if there is any numbness, pins and needles or tingling. Check for altered sensation: with their eyes closed, can the victim feel you gently stroking their fingers or toes? Can they identify where you are touching? Can they differentiate between blunt and sharp touch?

- **M = *Movement.*** Loss of range of movement, weakness or paralysis means possible damage to nerves, the spine, muscles, tendons, ligaments, bones or joints. Check that they can move their fingers and toes in all the usual directions to the full range of movement.

- **S = *Strength.*** Is there any weakness when they try to move against your counter pressure or squeeze your hand? Compare with the other uninjured side.

Note: once a splint or compression bandage is applied, check regularly over the next 48 hours for any onset or increase in numbness, pins and needles, tingling, pain, loss of movement or change in colour. If there is any reduction in CSMS, loosen/remove the splint or bandage and re-apply.

Checking the vital signs

Vital signs consist of: pulse rate, respiratory rate, consciousness, temperature, skin colour and hydration, pupil size.

The vital signs reflect the victim's condition (getting worse, staying the same, getting better) and help decide on treatments and course of action. The vital signs should be taken and recorded at least every 15 minutes by your watch until the victim's condition is stable, then hourly until stable again, and then 4-hourly ('**stable**' means 4 consecutive recordings are the same, or improving).

Pulse rate
Count the number of heartbeats per minute. Is the pulse regular/irregular, strong/weak? The arterial pulse can be felt at the wrist, groin (femoral pulse) or the neck (carotid pulse).

Respiratory/breathing rate
Count the number of breaths per minute (a good way to do this, so their breathing remains natural, is to continue holding their wrist, pretending to take the pulse, but discreetly counting the breaths). Is it regular or irregular, deep or shallow, wheezy? Can the victim talk in normal sentences (see Asthma)?

Level of consciousness – 'AVPU' scale
There are many causes for a deteriorating level of consciousness and it is important to be able to have some idea over time if the victim is worse, stable or improving. The AVPU scale is a simple method of measuring the victim's level of consciousness in a remote situation.

A – Alert and oriented
The victim's knowledge of their situation reflects their degree of alertness.

(A × 4) = the victim can tell you: their name; the place; the time; and what happened

(A × 3) = the victim can only give you 3 of the above facts

(A × 2) = the victim can only give you 2 of the above facts

(A × 1) = the victim can only give you 1 of the above facts.

V – Verbal
The victim responds only to a loud verbal stimulus (eg 'Hello can you hear me?') with a groan, grimace, grunt, or they recoil from the noise.

P – Pain
They respond only to a painful stimulus (eg a pinch on the earlobe, arm or leg) by some movement.

U – Unresponsive
There is no response at all to any of the above.

Skin
Check the colour inside the victim's lower eyelid (or gums). This is normally pink (it goes pale or blue when shock is present, and possibly brick red in CO poisoning). Check their skin temperature (normally warm) and moistness (normally dry) by touching the victim's forehead with the back of your hand.

Temperature
If the skin feels hot or an infection is suspected, take their temperature with a thermometer.

VITAL SIGNS AT REST (approximate values, resting at sea level)
(Note: at high altitude, pulse and breathing rate increase compared to sea level)

	Normal	Abnormal	Shock developing
PULSE RATE	• 50–80 beats per min (children: 80–100) • regular • strong	• less than 50, more than 100 • irregular • weak, bounding	• 100 or more, hard to feel • becoming irregular • weak
RESPIRATORY RATE	• 12–20 breaths per min (children: up to 30) • regular • deep (children's breathing is shallower)	• less than 12, more than 20 • irregular • shallow, wheezy, noisy etc	• 25 or more • becoming fast, irregular • shallow
LEVEL OF CONSCIOUSNESS	Ax4	Ax3, Ax2, Ax1, V, P, U	decreasing
SKIN	• pink • dry • warm	• pale, red, white, bluish, grey • hot, cold, cool • sweating, clammy	• pale, bluish, grey • cool, sweating • clammy
TEMPERATURE	oral 35 to 36.5°C (rectal 37.2°C)	less than 35°C, more than 37°C	normal, or low (high in pneumonia, septicaemia)

PART 2: Accident and illness protocol

77

10. EVACUATION

Evacuation of a sick or injured person from a wilderness setting is a major undertaking, requiring careful consideration of the following points and the consequences of each decision:

- consider the extent and severity of the problem versus your skills and equipment
- is their condition likely to improve or deteriorate?
- could the victim safely carry on or self evacuate after treatment?
- can the victim cope with the situation?
- is the safety of the group put at risk? Concern for the victim must override the group's enjoyment, but not its safety
- where is the nearest rescue point (eg road or landing strip) located?
- time till help arrives versus time for you to evacuate them yourself
- weather, distance and terrain to be traversed
- how will you let rescuers know if you have to change your plans?

Having thought and talked all this through with the victim and the group as appropriate, decide what to do: stay put and wait for rescue, carry out the evacuation yourself, or start moving in the direction of an approaching rescue team. You must continuously re-assess the situation to factor in any changed circumstances. All this requires good leadership skills and informed involvement of your group or team.

Sending for help

A rescue request requires the information indicated in Appendix 3.

If you don't have them ask about and search for radios and telephones (usually available at national park headquarters, police or army posts). Enquire about medical personnel, health posts or hospitals in the area where you are. A map of the area and/or GPS coordinates are essential, and a mud map helps. Put yourself in the position of the rescuers: how will they know where you are? What do they need to know?

- Rescue requests can be sent by messenger (send at least two people if possible), radio, telephone or satellite phone, and are usually sent to only one search and rescue organization.
- If you are alone, wait before leaving to get help until the victim is conscious, stable and all conditions are treated. Leave a dated note of your

name and intended route with the victim and mark your route (eg using broken branches, scraps of clothing).

Good communication

This needs careful thought and training.

- Make sure to practise on the devices chosen before departure. Make test calls to verify connections.
- VHF and mobile phones are line of sight (transmission and the signal strength is reduced by your head, foliage especially when wet, and vehicles, so be prepared to move). Sat phones don't work in ravines. SMS messages may get through when voice does not. HF works better at night.
- Transmission: write down your message, prioritizing the information order. Speak clearly in a higher than normal pitch of voice. Deliver message in short sections and ask 'copy so far?' to confirm receipt. If no response, keep trying; you may get through later or the receiving station may actually be hearing you. 'Over' means you are stopping transmitting and are waiting for a reply. 'Out' means you have finished your transmission.
- Record all your calls and communications.
- Signal your position or distress by means of shouts, whistles, gunshots (three distinct shouts, blasts, shots repeated), flares, smoke or fire.

Evacuating the victim

The leader/doctor should go with the victim if they are seriously ill or injured. Groups may have to abort their trip and return with the leader. Sick or injured people (especially local people and porters) should NEVER be sent back alone and the person going with them should understand the problem, speak the victim's language and have all the resources needed, including enough local money. Send with the victim a written copy of your record of what has happened, findings of the secondary survey and all treatments.

Means of evacuation

- Exhausted but conscious people may be '**towed**', either with a short rope around their waist as a leash, or by using walking poles, handheld or taped/tied to their belt or rucksack waist belt (tow from in front when going up, steady from behind when going down).

- A strong person may be able to **carry** a victim (conscious or unconscious), especially downhill. This is very efficient if a harness is improvised with ropes/slings/rucksack and two or more carriers work in short relays.
- Transporting a victim using **animals** (eg horses and yaks) can be efficient, but unsuitable for the unconscious or semiconscious.
- A **stretcher** carry is exhausting and will require 10 strong people over rough terrain. However, stretchers may be the only way to transport a victim with severe injuries or severe hypothermia.
- **Helicopter evacuation** may be necessary for a very ill or injured person.

Helicopter evacuation

In many countries, helicopters will only come if someone guarantees payment (possibly up to US$3000 per hour). They will want to see a proof of insurance, a credit card or cash. In some countries, including India and Pakistan, the army may be willing to provide a helicopter. In Tibet and many others countries, helicopter rescues are non-existent at the time of writing.

Landing a helicopter

- Select a large, flat, clear area, minimum size 30×30m. Trees may need to be cut down to open one side of a clearing. Tell everyone to stay well clear of this Landing Zone (LZ) except a small, selected 'helicopter team' who will help load the victim.
- Using white or coloured materials, construct a large 'H' in the LZ (minimum 6m across – but remove such materials before the helicopter lands to prevent it blowing up into the rotors) and/or make smoke to mark the site.
- One person should stand upwind of the 'H' with their back to the wind at the edge of the LZ, holding a scarf in their outstretched arm to indicate the ground wind direction to the pilot. Everyone else including the victim should be well behind this person, 30–40m from the LZ. The helicopter may circle a couple of times before landing.
- Once the helicopter has landed, wait until the pilot waves you forward. Approach the helicopter from the front (the pilot should be able to see you clearly) thus avoiding the rear rotor, and bend down as you do so, to avoid drooping main rotor. On sloping ground, approach up or across the slope. Turning rotor blades are invisible.
- Never wave at or signal a passing helicopter unless you have sent for one or desperately need one.
- The correct way to signal to a helicopter is shown in the diagram below.

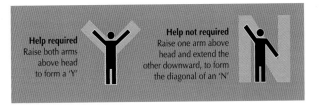

Help required
Raise both arms above head to form a 'Y'

Help not required
Raise one arm above head and extend the other downward, to form the diagonal of an 'N'

Fig 10.1 Signalling a helicopter

Helicopter rescue at sea

Having called for help, heave to, or at least slow your boat down by lying-a-hull or streaming warps, drogue or sea anchor. Be ready to illuminate your boat and deploy flares. The helicopter will usually make VHF contact. They appreciate some indication of wind direction and strength (smoke flare, flag). Rescues usually take place off the stern of the boat so clear this area of any removable obstructions.

Rescue techniques differ depending on the country. In most cases, the victim is placed in a sling and hoisted.

- One technique is for the victim to jump into the water, once instructed to do so, where they are plucked from the water by a rescuer on a wire.
- Another method is to send down a guideline to the boat (which must be held by hand and never attached to the boat); this is used to guide the rescuer to the deck of the boat.

IN CASE OF DEATH

Report (or send a report) to the police and ask them to inform the victim's next-of-kin and embassy. Do not move the body until the local police have given permission, as doing so can cause you a lot of trouble. Secure the victim's passport/ID card, insurance details, valuables, diary, camera and film. If you have to move the body (eg because of a risk of avalanche, flooding, wildlife scavenging, robbery), secure it by placing it in a groundsheet, tent fly or the victim's own sleeping bag, and if necessary bury and/or cover with stones. Photograph the whole process for the police, the victim's next-of-kin, and for legal and insurance purposes. If you have to leave the body unattended, mark the spot carefully and map and photograph the location so it can easily be found again. The victim's next-of-kin are the only people legally entitled to decide on how the body should finally be disposed of.

Allow members of your group time to say goodbye with prayers or a ceremony, if they so wish. Some may suffer from critical incident stress.

11. SPINAL AND HEAD INJURIES

Spinal injuries and head injuries (skull fractures, damage to the brain) are not common but are serious and best prevented. A thorough secondary survey is necessary to help determine the type and severity of an injury, while continuing observation will determine if improvement or deterioration is occurring.

Suspect injuries to the spine (neck or backbone), skull bones and brain in the following situations (the greater the speed involved, the greater the risk of significant injury):

- **accidents:** motor vehicle, horse riding, biking, skiing, speed boats, booms on yachts
- **falls:** especially of more than three times the victim's body height, especially if landing on head, back or buttocks
- **water:** jumping or diving, or being 'dumped' by waves or swept down a river rapid
- **blows** to the head, neck, shoulder or back, as may occur in fight
- **penetrating injuries** to the neck, chest or abdomen.

Note: when doing a primary survey in any of these situations, see 'Immobilization techniques', p. 33.

A decision may have to be made on whether the victim can start moving in order to self-rescue or continue with trip activities. The box 'Is this a serious spinal injury or can they move?' (below) will help you decide this. Refer to Chapters 2, 7, 8 and 9 as needed.

Specific injuries

Spinal (neck and backbone) injuries

Symptoms and signs

- The victim says to you, 'Don't move (or touch) me', 'There is something wrong with my head (neck or spine)', 'I can't move', 'I'm paralysed' or 'I can't feel my legs'
- The victim is semiconscious, unconscious or has been unconscious
- Fits (seizures)
- Loss of control of bowel or bladder (incontinence or failure to go)
- Developing signs of shock

- Deformity, swelling or significant wounds to head, neck, shoulders or back
- Pain, tenderness, soreness, numbness affecting the head, neck or anywhere along the back
- Pins and needles, or loss (or reduction) of sensation
- Muscles in arms or legs may be stiff, flaccid or weak

Treatment

- Try to keep the victim still and in the position found. However, if rescue/medical advice is unavailable and the position is too painful/awkward to maintain, or if it prevents vital treatment, you may gently try to straighten the victim's body out. Apply a steady gentle pull (traction) to the head in the direction it is pointing, and turn their face so it looks forward. Now move the head across until it is in line with the body, aiming to support the head manually in a natural, neutral position. Stop if pain occurs.
- If the victim is conscious and can swallow normally, nurse them on their back. If the victim is unconscious, use a spinal roll to put them in the safe airway position. **Note:** neck splints (cervical collar) are NOT routinely used in remote settings, as the dangers usually outweigh the benefits, and backboards are only routinely used for extraction from vehicles.

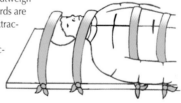

- Spinal lift or slide the victim onto a well-padded stretcher (use air mats, vacuum mats) prepared with suitable padding for the natural curves of the back and neck.

Fig 11.1 Makeshift spinal stretcher

- Secure them with sufficient padding, bandages and strapping firm enough so the stretcher can be turned on its side if vomiting occurs.
- Continue recording vital signs.

Note: long periods of immobility can produce pressure sores.

IS THIS A SERIOUS SPINAL INJURY OR CAN THE VICTIM MOVE?

In a non-remote setting, serious spinal injuries are usually excluded through hospital investigations. However, in a remote setting it may be necessary to decide if the injured person can start moving due to imminent danger, absence of rescue etc. Here is a protocol to help make this often-difficult decision:

- Repeat (or carry out) the secondary survey to find if the following points can be confirmed:
  - the victim IS conscious, alert and orientated to time and place (AVPU = Ax4)
  - they are NOT under the influence of alcohol or drugs
  - there are NO other painful injuries that could be a distraction
  - there is NO pain or tenderness when applying gentle pressure on each single bony prominence (vertebral spine) of the entire neck and back
  - CSMS is normal in all (uninjured) limbs
  - there is NO numbness around the buttocks or genital area

- If any of these points above are NOT confirmed, or if pain or loss or abnormality of sensation/movement/strength occurs, maintain full spinal injury precautions .

- If ALL points above are confirmed, ask the victim to start moving their limbs, body and neck, one part at a time (they should do this themselves; do not assist them). If this still does not cause pain or loss of sensation/movement/strength, they may start moving.

Significant head (skull and brain) injury

Significant blows to the head, including the face, may cause damage to the brain, internal bleeding or increased **intracranial pressure (ICP**: this is a general swelling of the brain due to severe internal jarring and bruising). Broken skull bones, including those of the ear and of the face (sinuses and eye sockets), may lead to infection reaching the brain. All these problems share similar symptoms and treatments, and need urgent evacuation. With all significant head injuries remember the possibility of neck injury.

Bleeding is more likely if the victim has been taking blood thinning medication, aspirin or NSAIDs.

Symptoms and signs
One or more of the following signs or symptoms may be present or appear later (in some cases up to a week later):
- changed behaviour: irritability, lethargy, withdrawal, confusion
- short term memory loss
- severe persistent headache, nausea or vomiting
- blurred or double vision: pupils not reacting to light or unequal in size
- increasing clumsiness (ataxia: see Finger–nose test, p. 168), slurred speech
- fits (seizures)
- increasing paralysis or numbness and weakness of the limbs or face
- deteriorating level of consciousness
- unconsciousness (often accompanied by noisy or irregular breathing).

Treatment
- Apply spinal precautions, with special attention to the neck.
- Strong painkillers are not usually given in head injuries as they may cause drowsiness or mask worsening condition but, in a remote setting, they may be needed if the victim is agitated and distressed by pain.
- Evacuate urgently.

Fractured skull
Breaks may occur anywhere in the skull but remember facial injuries often involve skull fractures. Infection of the brain may occur if the fracture is 'open'.

Symptoms and signs
- Any of the above symptoms of significant brain injury
- Dents, irregularities or wounds in the bones of the skull, or a 'crunchy' or 'boggy' sensation when gently feeling the skull bones
- With a fracture to the base of the skull there may be:
  ‣ bruising behind the ears ('Battle's sign') or around the eyes ('Racoon eyes')
  ‣ clear (spinal) fluid or blood draining from an (uninjured) nose or ear (signs of an open fracture)
  ‣ facial injuries.

Treatment
- If there is bleeding from the fracture site and the victim is conscious, support the neck then prop the victim up so their head is raised (if on a stretcher, raise the head end by 30°) and wait. If life-threatening bleeding doesn't stop, apply pressure around the fracture site using a ring pad.
- Clean and cover all wounds: see Chapter 14.
- Facial injuries can interfere with the airway: nurse the victim face down.
- If the fracture is open (on the scalp, ear or face via the nasal sinuses or around the eye socket), infection may reach the brain. Start antibiotics as for open fracture (Appendix 2).

Concussion
This is a milder form of brain injury when a blow to the skull jars and bruises the brain tissues but there is no raised intracranial pressure or significant symptoms.

Symptoms and signs
- There may be a brief episode of unconsciousness/semi-consciousness for a minute or two
- Short-term memory loss and disorientation: 'what happened?'
- Headache which may persist, dizziness
- Persistent tiredness, depression

Note: these symptoms should usually improve within 48 hours and disappear within a week, but headaches may persist on and off for weeks afterwards.

Treatment
- Rest and check vital signs 2-hourly for 24 hours.
- Give paracetamol for headache (do NOT give aspirin or NSAIDs, which may cause bleeding in the brain).
- Remember that serious problems may develop days later, so keep an eye on the victim for a week.

12. BURNS

Burns may be caused by flames, hot objects, hot fluids, air or gases, chemicals, lightning or the sun. Extensive burns, with pain and fluid loss (either from burned skin or into tissues causing swelling or blisters), may cause shock. Adequate pain relief through cooling, covering and painkillers is vital. The kidneys may stop working due to fluid loss and the airway may be threatened by damage to face, throat, trachea or lungs by hot air or smoke.

> **DEFINITIONS**
> - **Superficial burns:** skin is red or pale without blisters and is painful
> - **Partial thickness burns:** skin is red or discoloured, with blisters. Sensation is present varying from a sense of pressure to very painful
> - **Full thickness burns:** white or blackened skin with no blisters, no sensation, no pain

Burn management

Emergency treatment
- Remove from the heat source. If clothing is on fire: stop the victim moving around, drop them to the ground, cover with a blanket, coat etc and/or roll them to put out the flames.
- Cool the burn immediately with water (even if not drinkable): put the burnt part in water, run water over it (or apply water compresses) for 20 minutes. Room temperature water is preferable to cold (which may cause hypothermia). Water cooling is effective even if started up to half an hour after the burn occurred. Do NOT use ice.
- Chemical burns should be continuously flushed with water for at least 20 minutes.
- Remove rings, watches, jewellery and loose non-adherent clothing (which retains heat).
- Keep the victim warm by covering unburnt areas to prevent hypothermia.
- Give adequate pain relief (start with an NSAID eg ibuprofen, naproxen or diclofenac, then add other non-NSAID painkillers as needed) as soon as possible.
- Shock will occur in burns to more than 20% of body surface. Start shock prevention and stabilization.

Burns that require evacuation

With scrupulous wound care, adequate dressing material and painkillers, it is possible to treat a non-infected partial thickness burn of up to 5% of total body surface area in a wilderness setting. The following burns will require evacuation:

- burns (other than the most superficial or small) to face, hands, feet or perineum (between the legs, around the anus and genitals) and burns that encircle a limb
- partial thickness burns of more than 5% of total body surface area
- full thickness burns
- chemical burns (battery acid, kerosene etc)
- electrical burns, including lightning strike
- smoke inhalation injury (see below)
- burns on babies or small children
- infected burns or burns where infection is more likely (inner thigh, groin, around the genitals, anus and buttocks)
- when pain/dehydration cannot be controlled
- when other serious injuries are present (broken bones etc)
- when you, or the victim, cannot cope.

ESTIMATING THE SIZE OF A BURN

Only partial and full thickness burns are considered when estimating burn size.

Rule of Nines (used for adults)

- Head and neck = 9% (of total body surface area)
- Chest and abdomen = 18%
- Back = 18%
- Arms = 9% each
- Legs = 18% each
- Genital area (perineum) = 1%

Rule of Palms (used for babies, children and small burns on adults)

The size of the victim's palm is about 1% of their total body surface area. Use the size of their palm to estimate the percentage of the body burnt.

Cleaning a burn

- To reduce the risk of infection, all instruments should be cleaned (see 'Cleaning instruments' p. 110) and dressings should be sterile. Make sure the water used for cleaning burns does not drain away over nearby burns (especially drainage from around the buttocks).
- Remove all burnt clothing and material unless it is stuck to the burn, in which case trim round it.
- Clean the burn gently but thoroughly with drinkable water at room temperature, then dry it carefully.
- If the burn is very dirty, clean with povi-iodine solution 1% or other disinfectant solution, and finish with drinkable water.

Covering (dressing) a burn

The aim is to keep the burn moist (but not wet) with its own uninfected (ie clear) fluid (exudate) and prevent infective contamination. In the first few hours there will be lots of exudate, which will gradually decrease. Excluding air from the burn reduces pain.

- If the burn is absolutely clean, cover with a sterile non-stick (preferably permeable) dressing, eg special burn dressings (Aquagel™, Tegapore™, or Melolin™, Opsite™, Telfa™) or clear plastic food wrap (ClingWrap™, Saran Wrap™). Do not use plain gauze as it sticks to burns.
- If an infection starts, use an antiseptic burn cream (eg silver sulfadiazine) or an antibiotic cream. Pure honey or plain sugar, made into a thick paste by stirring in a few drops of drinkable water, makes an emergency antibacterial paste. Apply the cream (or paste) to a non-stick dressing, then place on the burn. Cover with a sterile non-stick dressing.
- Now add clean absorbent padding (gauze, cotton wool, sanitary pads, nappies) over the non-stick dressing, loosely held in place with bandages.
- Change the dressings when they are soaked with exudate, which will be frequently to start with, then at least every day.
- If old dressings are stuck to the burn, soak them off with warm drinkable water. Take your time (up to 20 minutes) as this can be painful: pain relief may be needed.
- Blisters should be left alone, unless they are broken, in which case remove the skin.
- Once burns are dry (no more exudate, or the amount is decreasing) and not infected, pure aloe vera gel can be applied.

PART 3: Problems and their treatment

Ongoing treatment
- Once burns are cleaned and covered, start giving liquid replacement (see 'Type of rehydration liquid', p. 144). Large burns will require large volumes.
- Elevate the burned part to reduce swelling.
- If infection develops, treat as for wound infection. Tetanus is a possibility, so check vaccination status.
- The medically trained can insert a urinary catheter for burns around the genital area.

Specific burns

Burns to hands and feet
- Separate fingers and toes with non-stick dressings and cover as explained above.
- Cover with a plastic bag secured at the wrists or ankles with adhesive tape, or wrap in plastic food wrap.
- Encourage movement of fingers or toes when pain allows.

Smoke inhalation injury
Burns can be complicated by having breathed in flames, fumes or hot smoke. If the victim was exposed to smoke in a confined space or have burns to face, lips, nostrils or eyebrows, assume smoke inhalation injury is present. There may also be CO poisoning.

The signs are: rapid, difficult or noisy breathing, 'brassy' cough, hoarse voice. The victim may appear reasonable initially but may deteriorate later.
- Sit them up and give oxygen (8L/min).
- Evacuate urgently.

Sunburn
- Apply cold compresses.
- Painkillers may be needed for the first 24 hours or so.
- Apply aloe vera gel 8-hourly.

13. BROKEN BONES, DISLOCATIONS, SPRAINS AND STRAINS

In a wilderness setting it doesn't matter whether you know exactly what the injury is, which is often impossible anyway; simply doing the basics well is sufficient. What you need to work out is one of three possibilities:

- Can the victim carry on with the trip?
- Will the trip have to be modified to cope with the injury?
- Does the victim need evacuation?

DEFINITIONS

- **Break, crack, fracture:** different words for damage to a bone

- **Dislocation:** the bones at a joint are displaced from their normal position

- **Closed fracture:** the skin is not broken

- **Open (compound) fracture:** the bones are in contact with the outside through a break (wound) in the skin, however small or hidden (eg in the nose or ear)

- **Angulated fracture:** the broken bones are pushed out of their normal shape

- **Sprains:** injuries to joints where the supporting ligaments are stretched, partially torn or completely torn; most sprains occur at the wrist, ankle, knee and thumb joints

- **Strains:** tearing or bruising injuries of a muscle mass or tendon due to sudden stretching when the muscle is contracting during movement, from lifting with poor posture, or sometimes from a direct, crushing blow

- **Complicated injury:** injuries where there is a mixture of the above injuries and/or damage to nerves or blood vessels

- **Traction:** a steady continuous pull applied to both ends of a broken bone (or limb) in order to overcome muscle spasm, relieve pain and straighten the broken/dislocated bone into its correct position

- **Reduction:** straightening a deformed limb using traction to relocate a fracture/dislocation back into its normal position

---

General considerations

- Determine the mechanism of injury (MOI – see p. 49) and perform a thorough physical examination in your secondary survey, as this will help determine severity, likely location and type of injury.
- The commonest injuries are to wrist and ankle due to tripping or falling. From the point of view of immediate treatment of these injuries, it doesn't matter whether it is broken or not. Minor soft tissue injuries and sprains usually settle quite quickly and the victim may be able to continue the trip. Fractures will not settle quickly. Do not worry about 'missing a fracture' as those that need immediate specific treatment and evacuation will be obvious.
- In a wilderness setting most injuries are likely to be restricted to one or two sites, in which case shock is unlikely: vehicle accidents and long, high speed falls are the exception. Shock is more likely with multiple injuries.
- Always check for CSMS (at least circulation and sensation – checking movement may be impractical) below the injury site every 30 minutes. You may not be able to find a pulse, but you can assess circulation (see 'Checking CSMS', p. 74).
- Loss of CSMS below the injury means an attempt must be made to straighten a break or reduce a dislocation within two hours as there is risk of permanent damage.
- Early, effective pain relief is important.
- Be wary of younger children, the elderly and the obese: they break differently and more easily.

General management

Closed fractures

Symptoms and signs
- There can be obvious symptoms and signs: a 'snapping' sensation or even sound at the time of the injury, immediate onset of pain, deformity (change in shape, compare with uninjured limb), a feeling or sound of crackling or grating on touching and moving the fracture site.
- Swelling at the injury site occurring quickly (within 1 or 2 hours or even quicker) implies bleeding into the injury. This usually implies a significant injury that will need evacuation. Swelling that occurs more slowly, perhaps overnight implies an inflammatory reaction and may indicate less severity.

- Usually there is tenderness and some loss of function (such as decreased grip strength in a wrist or unable to stand on an ankle).

Treatment
- Initially keep the victim still, in the 'position found'.
- Immediately support the injured limb/part in the position found by holding it with your hands, an assistant's hands and/or the victim's hands to prevent further injury and help ease pain.
- Give adequate pain relief including ice or cold water compresses, and continue shock prevention and stabilization.
- Carry out a thorough secondary survey, paying special attention to CSMS.
- Attempt to straighten the limb (reduction), especially if CSMS is compromised or evacuation is delayed, and apply a splint.
- See specific injuries below.

Open fractures

Symptoms and signs
- The signs of a closed fracture are present, but with bone obviously exposed or even protruding from the skin.
- Wounds over a fracture site may be the only indication that the fracture is open, especially round the face, eyes and ears.
- Partial amputations and crush injuries (p. 121) involve open fractures.

Treatment
These are less common than closed fractures and require additional management and urgent evacuation, as the risk of permanent damage from infection is high. The general principles for closed fractures apply, plus the following:
- clean the wound; treat as an open wound and cover with a sterile dressing
- after checking CSMS attempt to straighten (reduce) the limb
- apply a splint, which should allow access for ongoing wound care if evacuation is delayed
- start antibiotics as soon as possible (Appendix 2).

See specific injuries below.

Dislocations

Symptoms and signs
- Dislocation of a joint may be simple, or complicated by a fracture.

- There is loss of function, change of shape and possible changes to CSMS beyond the injury.

Treatment

Dislocations should be reduced as soon as possible, especially if there is abnormal CSMS beyond the injury. Make a note of CSMS before and after attempting a reduction. Reduction usually improves CSMS. Even if reduction is successful, all victims with dislocations should be followed up by a doctor as there may be undiagnosed associated fractures that must be treated. See specific injuries below.

Sprains

Symptoms and signs

These commonly occur at wrist, ankle and knee when the ligaments are stretched or torn. The joint is swollen, tender and painful.

Treatment

Give rest, compression, elevation and cold treatment, followed by strapping and sometimes a splint. Do not apply heat. See specific injuries below.

Strains

Symptoms and signs

The commonest strains are to the back, groin, thigh and calf. Pain and swelling may occur, internal bleeding of the muscle is common and may result in a collection of blood (**haematoma**) in the muscle. There may be marked loss of function but little or no loss of CSMS.

Treatment

Strains are best treated by keeping the damaged muscle moving (although total bed rest may be needed for a day or two, followed by gradual mobilization), keeping warm and encouraging good posture. Gentle massage, liniment and local heat after 48 hours (improvised heat pack/hot water bottle) may help, and painkillers (maximum dose of ibuprofen, with paracetamol or codeine if needed) may be necessary. Diazepam (2.5mg 8 to 12-hourly) is useful for severe muscle spasm. Sprains usually recover spontaneously over days.

Multiple injuries

Symptoms and signs

These are obvious and caused by large amounts of force, typically motor vehicle accidents or long/high speed falls. Shock is likely.

Treatment

Follow the accident illness protocol. Assume until proven otherwise there are more injuries that you can see, especially to internal organs. Place the victim carefully and securely on a stretcher using spinal precautions and pelvic splinting. The victim should not be given food, but may be given water if there will be a delay of at least 6 hours before getting to hospital.

REDUCING FRACTURES

There are three principles for reducing fractures: pain relief, persistent adequate traction, and patience.

- Fractures with altered sensation or circulation beyond the break must be reduced within two hours of the injury.

- Other fractures can be reduced to improve pain, splinting, bleeding or movement.

- Don't be surprised if you find it difficult and unpleasant for you and the victim.

- Do your best: you are not going to make the injury worse, but you may make it better. Any victim with an injury that has prompted you to consider reduction should be evacuated urgently.

How to apply traction

Inform the victim that the process may be painful and get their consent. While there is a short time after the accident when the break is 'numb' and reducing can sometimes be carried out without painkillers, in most cases strong painkillers (Penthrox™ or fentanyl lozenges are a good option for wilderness procedures) or local/general anaesthetics will be necessary.

- Instruct helpers to hold the victim's broken limb (or body) above the fracture and to be ready to apply counter-traction when you apply traction at the other side of the break (if the angulation is

97

severe, another helper should support the broken area – using a broad sling – so that straightening does not occur until the broken ends are drawn apart).

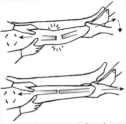

- Take hold of the limb or digit below the injury with both hands, and slowly but firmly start pulling that part in the direction it is pointing. This will gradually overcome the muscle spasm around the break and draw the broken

Fig 13.1 Straightening an angulated lower leg fracture

ends of the bone apart. This may take several minutes. **Note:** the pain should decrease: if it becomes unbearable, stop, splint as is and evacuate urgently.

- Now, while maintaining traction, gently move the bone back into its correct position and splint.

- Once splinted, check that CSMS is present. If CSMS is lost or worse after straightening the limb, restore the part to a position in which CSMS is as normal as possible and splint in that position.

See also specific injuries below.

SPLINTING

Splinting is any technique used to keep a broken bone, dislocated joint, sprained or injured part completely still. Splinting may be applied to a limb, digits, the spine, ribs, collarbones or pelvis. Don't get too concerned about specific types of splints for specific fractures. Use common sense and aim for the position of most comfort or, in reality, position of least discomfort!

- A good splint reduces pain, bleeding and further damage to tissues by jagged ends of broken bones. Splinting prepares the victim for evacuation (or other procedures). A good splint has normal CSMS beyond the injury site and the victim feels much better.

- The aim is to apply something rigid (the 'splint'), placed alongside the injury and held in place by bandages or sling. A sling or even a stretcher may be needed to finish immobilizing the part.

- There is a wide range of manufactured splints available. SAM™ splints are cheap, multi-functional and reusable, and ideal for wilderness travel. Vacuum splints are excellent but bulkier and more expensive. Lightweight traction splints are available for broken thighbones. Avoid inflatable splints as they can compromise CSMS.

- Improvised splints can be made from closed cell or inflatable sleeping mats, backpacks (or parts of), skis, ski/tent poles, canoe paddles, doors, the uninjured leg etc. When folded into a 'gutter', cardboard or a sleeping mat becomes quite rigid. A large roll of duct tape and plastic food wrap (ClingWrap™) are invaluable when improvising splints.

Applying a splint

To be effective, a splint must *completely stop* any movement at the fracture/dislocation site *and* of the (uninjured) joints above and below the injury.

- Remove rings, jewellery, watches and clothing within the splint area.

- Place limbs in the 'position of comfort': wrist in a neutral position, knee slightly bent, elbows and ankles bent at 90°.

- Insert padding (eg cotton wool, towels, T-shirts, sweaters, sanitary pads) between the splint and the limb. This must fill natural and unnatural gaps between the limb and the splint. Padding prevents pressures sores, which are especially likely when bone is close to the skin surface (eg wrists, ankles, elbows). Avoid creases or lumps in the padding, which must be soft and smooth.

- Check CSMS below the splint every 30 minutes for the first 48 hours. Instruct the victim to tell you of any increasing pain or numbness. If this does occur (CSMS is decreasing or lost), or pain is starting, undo the splint and re-apply less tightly once CSMS has returned to normal.

- If the splint does not reduce pain/improve comfort, examine for other injuries and/or improve and re-apply the splint.

PART 3: Problems and their treatment

Specific injuries

Fingers/toes

A broken or dislocated finger/toe is usually easy to spot and equally easy to reduce with traction, as there are no big muscles to overcome. Splint by taping it to its neighbour (with some absorbent material between them); add a wrist splint if necessary.

Hand

Broken bones in the hands most commonly occur from a crush or a punch-type injury. Telling the difference between just severe bruising and one or more breaks may be difficult. In the short term it doesn't matter. Use ice to reduce swelling and splint in a position of comfort with plenty of padding. Splint as for wrist below.

Wrist

Wrist injuries are common and may range from a sore wrist to an obviously deformed broken wrist which should be reduced if possible.

Test the grip strength of the victim by asking them to squeeze your hand, test mobility by asking them to do a 'thumbs up', and finally test for tenderness by pressing gently on the bony parts of the wrist. Bony tenderness, weak grip and inability to do a thumbs up suggests a fracture.

Whether it is a bad sprain or a break, apply a splint along the palm side of the forearm and wrist, from the elbow to the knuckles. Curl the fingers around the well-padded end of the splint with the wrist bent slightly back (if this is comfortable).

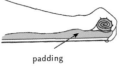

padding

Place in a broad arm sling with the forearm slightly elevated. Exercise the fingers regularly.

Fig 13.2 Forearm and wrist splint

Forearm

Fractures in the forearm usually involve both bones and result in an unstable, wobbly arm. Reduce and splint as for wrist.

Elbow

Injuries usually occur from over-extending the joint, a direct blow to the pointy bit at the back of the joint, or a twisting fall onto it with rotation of the forearm.

PART 3: Problems and their treatment

In a normal elbow the three pointy bits at the back form a straight line when the arm is straight out and an equal sided triangle when fully bent; this arrangement is lost in a dislocation. A dislocated elbow may contain a fracture as well: either way it will look weirdly deformed and will need reduction as soon as possible.

To reduce it, gently straighten the elbow whilst applying traction. With an assistant 'bear hugging' the victim (including the injured arm) to provide counter-traction, progressively increase the force along the line of the arm. This may require a lot of force. If this does not succeed, place your other forearm in the crook of the victim's fore-arm, close to the elbow, and use it to continue providing traction and as a fulcrum while you decisively bend the elbow joint. This will usu-ally work.

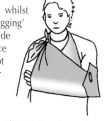

Fig 13.3 Broad arm sling

If it is painful but not deformed, it still may be broken. Put in a broad arm sling.

Upper arm
Fractures along the bone of the upper arm are very painful and result in a deformed, unstable, wobbly arm. Apply a collar and cuff sling then bandage the arm to the chest or wear clothing over it.

Shoulder girdle (shoulder, shoulder blade, collarbone)
Injuries usually result from a fall onto an outstretched hand or falling onto the shoulder. Another cause of dislocation is in paddle sports, when the arm is forced up and behind the head. Additionally, there may be some twisting component. Injuries may also occur from direct blows to the injured part, either being struck with something, or for example by falling onto the shoulder. Injuries in two places are uncom-mon but do occur.

Look at and feel for swelling, tenderness or deformity suggestive of a fracture: the place where the collar bone attaches to the sternum (breast bone), the collar bone itself, where the collar bone attaches to the shoulder blade (a common site of injury), the shoulder itself (where a depression rather than the usual rounded shape suggests a dislocation – with the arm held out to the side by the victim), the shoulder blade, and finally check down the bone of the upper arm.

A **broken collar bone** may be helped by bandages around the shoulder, which are then tied tightly together across the back, in order to brace the shoulders back.

All other injuries should be supported/splinted in a position of comfort.

A **dislocated shoulder** should be reduced as soon as possible: the longer it is out, the harder it is to get back. Some people have recurrent shoulder dislocations and know exactly what has happened to them and some know how to fix it. Check for numbness on the

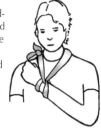

Fig 13.4 Collar and cuff sling

arm just below the dislocation. If there is altered sensation or weakness, reduction is urgent (document your findings before and after reducing it).

REDUCING A DISLOCATED SHOULDER

There are many methods for reducing a dislocated shoulder. Here are three that are safe and easy to perform. They require time and patience.

- **Method 1:** Place the victim face down on a flat(ish) surface, such as a table or log. Encourage the injured arm to hang down vertically. The victim should hold a small weight (3–5kg) in their hand to encourage reduction. This may take 10–20 minutes.

- **Method 2:** Lie the victim on their back and encourage the injured arm to come down to the side (it will…even if it doesn't look like it!). Kneel next to the injured side of the victim and gently grasp their hand. Keeping the arm straight, and applying some traction, very gently and very slowly lift up the arm until it is vertical. This process should take 5 minutes at least.

- **Method 3:** The following method is for reducing your own shoulder dislocation. Sit on the ground with your knees drawn up. Using your good hand, encourage the injured arm up so that you can grasp your hands around knees. Gently lean back – the combination of upper body weight and the resistance of your hands clasping your knees will apply traction. Again, this must be done very slowly and smoothly.

Feet

Telling the difference between just severe bruising and one or more breaks may be difficult. In the short term it doesn't matter. Use ice to reduce swelling and splint in a position of comfort.

Ankle

These are very common injuries, typically resulting from a 'twisted ankle', 'going over on it' or a fall from a height. There are many different types of fracture and sprains but the approach is the same: check CSMS, full range of normal movement, strength and weight bearing ability in order to assess the severity of the injury.

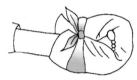

Fig 13.5 U-shaped blanket roll splint for ankle or foot

When an ankle is deformed and swells immediately after the accident, it will need pain relief, reduction (if there is any loss of CSMS), splinting (eg U-shaped blanket roll splint) and urgent evacuation.

Anything else is less urgent and is probably a sprain or stable minor fracture.

Painful ankles that swell up within a few hours or overnight and have tenderness on pressing the bones, will need pain relief, splinting and rest. These ankles will need to be x-rayed in a few days.

If the victim can walk a minimum of four steps on the injured ankle, it is most likely a sprain; if they cannot walk four steps, treat as a fracture. Sprains will gradually improve (and the victim will be able to carry on with good strapping) while a fracture will not.

Less severe injuries will improve over a day or two and improve quicker with mobilization and strapping.

STRAPPING A SPRAINED ANKLE

- Shave, clean and dry the lower leg.
- With the victim sitting with their injured leg straight out in front of them, put a loop of bandage around the toes and ask them to pull gently on it to hold their foot up.

- Apply 'stirrups' of adhesive non-stretch tape, starting on the side away from the injury down one side of the leg, under the heel and up the other side (tilt the ankle joint to the injured side, as you do so, to gain maximum support from the strapping).

- Hold the top ends of the stirrups in place with a spiral of tape (the spiral prevents constriction of the calf).

- Tape a U-shaped piece of closed cell mat around the anklebone on the injured side to control further swelling.

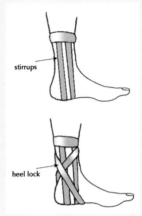

Fig 13.6 Strapping

- Apply a light pressure bandage over the strapping, from toes to knee.

- Exercise the thigh (leg raises to front and back, sets of 50, 4 times daily minimum) until walking.

- Once walking, add heel locks over the strapping (these prevent re-injury).

- Strapping is left in place for one to three weeks.

Lower leg (tibia and fibula shaft)

Broken bones in the lower leg above the ankle are always obvious, unstable and extremely painful. They often result from a twisting force up the leg whilst the lower part of the leg is restrained – eg skiing or a foot down a

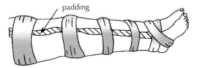

Fig 13.7 Leg-to-leg splint for thigh, knee, lower leg

hole. Pain relief, splint in the position of most comfort (eg using the good leg as a splint, using a closed cell mat) and evacuate urgently.

Knee

This is a cleverly designed and complex joint prone to several different injuries:

- A knee that blows up quickly is full of blood and has either a fracture or major ligament injury or both. Occasionally the victim can still weight bear, but usually they can't. Give pain relief, splint in a position of comfort, and evacuate urgently.

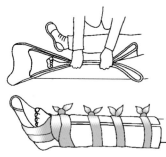

- A knee dislocation is very rare and should be treated as above. However, **dislocation of the kneecap** is not uncommon: bending and twisting results in sud-

Fig 13.8 Closed cell mat U-shaped gutter splint for lower leg or foot

den pain and the kneecap can be seen displaced out to the side as the victim holds the knee slightly flexed. Reduction is relatively easy: simultaneously lift and push the kneecap back while straightening the leg. The leg should be splinted straight and the victim is allowed to put weight on it. If walking is necessary, tape the kneecap away from the direction of dislocation.

- Twisting, compression or a combination of forces on the knee can result in various combinations of **injuries to ligaments and cartilage**. Accurate diagnosis is unlikely: if they can stand on it comfortably and still walk, don't worry too much – consider ice/cold water and a bandage, and re-assess the next day. If they cannot stand on it, use ice/cold water, elevation and pain relief. If it doesn't swell up overnight, it is unlikely to be serious. If it does, there is likely to be some damage that requires medical intervention, although not urgently.

- If the victim feels that their knee is unstable, wobbly and about to give way, they may have serious disruption to one or more ligaments. Splint with the knee slightly bent and evacuate.

- **Trekker's knee:** the knee becomes hot, swollen and painful without any specific history of injury or fever. It commonly occurs after several days of walking and especially after a long descent. If pain is severe, rest for a day or two, but bend the knee regularly (non-weight bearing). Apply anti-inflammatory cream and/or give painkillers (maximum dose of ibuprofen or naproxen). When walking, apply adhesive tape to the kneecap so that it is pulled slightly across toward the other knee. Warm up the joint before use, use a walking stick and avoid carrying any weight.

Thighbone (femur)

This bone is very strong and it takes big forces to break it. Activities where such injuries are likely are skiing/snowboarding, motorcycling, trail biking, in which case taking along a commercial traction splint (such as a CT6) might be advisable. Extreme pain, inability to stand and developing swelling in the thigh indicate a fractured femur. The leg may be shortened and rotated with the foot pointing outwards. Blood loss may be significant (1–1.5 litres), but the fit healthy adult will not go into shock if this is an isolated injury.

In a remote situation, if evacuation is not seriously delayed and especially if you don't have a commercial traction splint, a simple splint is sufficient. Splint the whole injured leg, either to the uninjured leg, or with a vacuum splint, or with improvised splinting. Splint in the position of most comfort. Evacuate by stretcher.

MAKING UP AN IMPROVISED TRACTION SPLINT

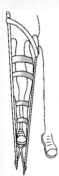

Fig 13.9 Traction splint for thigh or lower leg
Place an anchor round the top of the thigh (this can be a lumbar pad from a backpack, a life jacket, climbing harness etc). Attach suitable poles (eg walking/ski/tent poles, paddles) to the anchor on either side of the thigh. Now connect the victim's boot (use slings, tape or cut a hole through the leather in line with the leg bone and pass a sling through) to the end of the poles. Apply traction of about 10% of body weight using a 'Spanish windlass', mechanical ascender, rafting hitch or prusik knot. A rough guide to the amount of tension is a balance between pain relief at the break and uncomfortable pressure on the anchor at the top of the thigh.

A **traction splint** (see box for an improvised one) may be used if:

- there is no possibility of a pelvic fracture
- the other forms of splinting and painkillers are not relieving pain sufficiently
- there is no chance of evacuation within days or weeks
- the traction splint will not make evacuation more difficult due to its length.

Stop trying to apply a traction splint if it is causing too much pain. Improvised traction splints are not as easy to use as the commercial ones.

Hip

Hip fractures or dislocations are very painful and it is difficult to tell the difference between them. The victim will be unable to stand and there may be no visible swelling. Reducing either is unlikely. Provide pain relief, splint and evacuate urgently.

Pelvis

Pelvic fractures can be divided into two types: serious ones that are very rare and are associated with multiple injuries, and less obvious minor ones. If a high speed accident (car crash, long fall) is involved in which the victim has sustained other obvious injuries, particularly of the lower limbs, it is best to

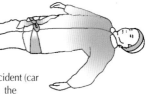

Fig 13.10 Splint for pelvis

assume that there is a significant pelvic fracture. In this case do not push on the pelvis but handle the victim carefully, leaving their clothes on. Using elastic bandages, strips of sheet or even belts, bind around the pelvis at hip level and NOT any higher, and not too tightly. Minor *stable* fractures of the pelvis may occur, however if there is any doubt treat as above.

A groin strain may resemble a minor fracture of the lower end of the pelvis, especially when the victim has fallen from a height and landed awkwardly. The victim with a groin strain can usually limp around, while one with a fracture cannot stand. If they can't stand, evacuate urgently; if they can stand, wait and re-assess.

Chest injuries

Chest injuries result from a fall or from a direct blow with a foreign object. Whether there are rib fractures or not is not important: what matters is whether there is damage to the underlying lung that impairs breathing. Pain relief is important, as pain can impair breathing.

107

Treatment

If there are no complications, give pain relief and use the arm on the injured side of the chest as a 'splint' by putting it into a broad arm sling with wide crepe bandages around the chest to reduce movement and support the injured side.

Complicated chest injury

If the underlying lung is damaged, the victim may be struggling for breath, breathing at rate greater than 25 breaths/min, coughing up blood, have blue lips or an open chest wound.

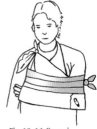

Fig 13.11 Broad arm sling and wide crepe bandages

- If individual **ribs** are broken in more than one place, an area of the chest wall may 'flail', ie the opposite to normal, moving in on inspiration and out on expiration. Place a large firm pad, such as a piece of closed cell sleeping mat, over the area and tape firmly in place.

- If there is a visible **sucking puncture wound** on the chest wall with red frothy bubbling blood/air, cover the wound with flexible plastic and seal on three sides to form a 'flap valve', allowing excess air/blood to escape (from the fourth, lower side) while preventing air being drawn in. Use tincture of benzoin, superglue or duct tape to hold the plastic in place.

A damaged lung may leak air into the chest cavity and the lung will collapse as the chest cavity on that side fills with air: this is a **pneumothorax**. If the leaking air becomes pressurized, a **tension pneumothorax** develops and breathing becomes difficult, neck veins swell and the trachea is pushed to the uninjured side. No air can be heard entering the collapsed lung and that side of the chest sounds hollow when tapped. If there is a chest wound gently push a gloved finger into it to release the air pressure. Dress the wound as above, without closing it (so air can escape).

A pneumothorax can also occur spontaneously, usually in tall, narrow-chested young men.

If there is a **penetrating object in the chest**, do not remove but wrap plastic food wrap around the base of the object; add plenty of padding and dressing, taping everything to the chest (but not all the way around their body if this interferes with their breathing). Then:

- Give oxygen (10 to 15L/min) or assisted breathing if the victim is blue or pale (see 'assisted breathing', p. 57).

- Encourage steady and even breathing, while discouraging excessive coughing (codeine can be used as a cough suppressant, but not if respiration is depressed).
- Nurse the victim sitting up if possible, having them support their damaged chest with their own hands. Lean them to, or lie them on, the injured side so internal bleeding pools away from uninjured lung.
- To prevent pneumonia, give enough painkillers to allow the victim to take 5 deep breaths and do some coughing every 30 minutes (supporting their injured chest with their hands as they do this). If a chest infection develops, give antibiotics as for pneumonia (Appendix 2).

Facial injuries

Victims with facial injuries may have an associated head or spinal injury. The face is well supplied with blood and even with minor injuries can swell up spectacularly. This may make it hard to decide if a fracture is present. If there is a fracture, pressing on bony parts away from the swelling will often cause pain.

- Airway protection is the first priority. Look carefully inside the nasal passages and mouth for damage, removing any broken teeth, blood etc.
- Sit the victim up with their head hanging down, use the recovery position or have them lying face down with the face supported as comfortably as possible. They must NOT be laid on their back.
- Facial fractures are often 'open', so give antibiotics as for open fracture (see Appendix 2). If the victim cannot swallow, empty the capsule contents, or crush tablets, and mix with something sweet (eg honey) to be sucked. Alternatively, the capsules can be given as suppositories or enema (see 'Ways to administer medications', p. 36).

Upper and lower jaw

Broken upper or lower jaws are especially dangerous, as blood, broken bone, loose teeth or a cut tongue may block the airway. Clear the airway, provide supporting bandages and evacuate.

Nose

A broken nose may be obviously bent after an injury. Act immediately: grip the nose firmly and straighten it out. This painful procedure should be quick and if you fail first time, don't persist; it can always be corrected once home. See 'Nosebleed', p. 123.

14. WOUNDS

Wounds include abrasions, cuts, flaps, puncture wounds, amputation (partial or complete), crush injuries and nosebleeds. Wounds may be life-threatening, with obvious or hidden injuries to bones, tendons, muscles, nerves, blood vessels, joints or vital organs. Good management prevents infection and maintains function.

The key to wound care is *control of bleeding, thorough cleaning* and *good dressing*.

General management

- In a wilderness setting, rapid control of significant bleeding is important and if direct pressure is initially insufficient, a temporary tourniquet may be used.
- Clean your instruments, wash your hands with soap and dry them. Wear surgical gloves, a mask/scarf and goggles/glasses (the latter especially while jet washing).
- Inspect the wound for damage and dirt, clean it to prevent infection and decide whether to leave it 'open' or to close it. If in doubt, leave open.
- Finally, cover (dress) the wound and give ongoing wound care.
- Splinting may be needed for comfort and to control bleeding.
- If blood loss is significant, give fluid replacement (see 'Type of rehydration liquid' p. 144).

CLEANING INSTRUMENTS

In a wilderness setting sterilization is usually impossible and a thorough cleaning is sufficient:

- scrub the instruments with a nailbrush in warm soapy water, rinse in drinkable water; then
- place in boiling water for 5 minutes OR soak in Dettol™ (1 tablespoon in 100ml water) for 10 minutes OR flame briefly with a lighter; then
- dry, preferably in the sun out of the wind; wrap in toilet paper (from a new roll) and place in ziplock bags.

ANAESTHETIZING A WOUND

These are various ways to reduce sensation around a wound before inspecting, cleaning, closing or dressing it:

- apply ice or snow (in a clean plastic bag) directly onto the wound and surrounding skin: this will decrease sensation for a short time
- apply topical anaesthetics (lidocaine gel) to abrasions or skin; wait 30 minutes before proceeding
- if trained, inject local anaesthetic into the surrounding tissue (but not into infected tissue) or give a regional block.

- Always check tetanus status and if needed (if more than 5 years since last vaccination) arrange for a course or a booster within 3 days.
- Evacuation is needed for significant blood loss, deep or dirty wounds, deep puncture wounds, loss of CSMS, crush injuries, deep puncture wounds, severe animal bites (if rabies/tetanus is a possibility), wounds needing debriding, if infection is uncontrollable, or if tetanus vaccination is needed.

Inspect the wound

- Lay out your instruments and dressings on a clean, dry surface.
- Anaesthetize the wound if pain prevents you from inspecting/cleaning it effectively.
- Look inside the wound with a good light and check for dirt, hair, foreign objects, any dead or dying tissue, or any damage to tendons, bones, nerves or internal organs.
- Test CSMS beyond the wound site.

Clean the wound

- Clip hair only if it is in the way or prevents good closure. Meticulously clear away all clippings and clean the skin around the wound with drinkable water, Savlon Dry™ spray, alcohol swabs, or **disinfectant solution** (eg povi-iodine 1%, or soapy drinkable water). Avoid getting disinfectant in the wound (if you do wash it out with drinkable water).
  - Abrasions: scrub clean with drinkable water, pick off any retained dirt then jet wash with drinkable water and dress.

111

- Clean wounds: small wounds (less than a centimetre, caused by a clean knife) don't need washing. Wash larger clean wounds with drinkable water.
- Dirty wounds (soil, clothing, debris etc): clean with disinfectant solution then jet wash with 1L of drinkable water. Pick out remaining dirt with tweezers and wash out again with drinkable water (use a jet wash if necessary). If it is still dirty, scrub clean with a gauze square while jet washing.
- Very dirty wounds (especially if there is soil, faecal matter, coral or sea water in it) or wounds caused by human or animal bites (especially if rabies is a possibility): scrub it as soon as possible with a gauze square and disinfectant solution (povi-iodine, soapy drinkable water etc) for two minutes by your watch. Then apply povi-iodine 1% solution to the wound for 5 minutes (if rabies is a possibility extend this to 30 minutes). Finally, thoroughly wash out the wound with drinkable water.
- Wounds with dead or dying skin, muscle or fat at the skin margins or in the wound must be debrided (below).
- Puncture wounds: allow, even encourage, bleeding for a few minutes then disinfect around it.
- In the hot tropics germs may be exotic (eg sea water and coral wounds) and infection particularly aggressive so even the smallest scratches, nicks, abrasions or bites need to be meticulously cleaned with disinfectant solution then covered and KEPT DRY.

Note: do NOT put antiseptic creams on open wounds as this promotes infection.

Leaving the wound 'open' or closing it?

Whether you decide to leave a wound 'open' or to close it, you must always cover it.

Closing a wound means bringing the cut surfaces together and holding them in place with closures (stitches, staples, adhesive strips or glue) until healed.

Leaving a wound 'open' means not using closures (but the edges may be brought approximately together by bandages).

A wound left 'open' has less chance of serious infection but takes longer to heal, may become infected and scars more than a 'closed' wound. Closing a wound with closures or stitches makes the wounded part more useful if the victim needs to walk, climb, paddle or sail to safety.

JET WASH

Fig 14.1 Jet wash

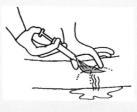

Jet washing means squirting drinkable water into a wound to clean it out. Use a large syringe (with a large needle or no needle) as a 'spray gun' to increase the pressure of the liquid. If you don't have a large (at least 10ml and preferably 50ml) syringe, use a clean strong plastic bag with a reinforced toothpick-sized hole in one corner, seal the top and squeeze; or use a hydration pack and its clean) tube. Use at least 200ml for a small wound (1L or more for larger or dirtier wounds).

DEBRIDING A WOUND

Debriding means removing obviously damaged tissue and/or foreign objects (woody splinters, clothing etc) from a wound. Debriding prevents infection (eg cellulitis, gas gangrene, tetanus), especially if muscle is damaged.

In the wilderness, debriding major wounds is carried out only if you have the necessary skills and evacuation is delayed by more than 48 hours (24 hours in the hot tropics), as there is risk of damage to vital structures.

- Anaesthetize the wound.
- Trim back all dead or dying tissue (bruised, discoloured, not bleeding) at the skin margins and especially inside the wound; trim back to viable tissue (pink/red and bleeding) using tweezers and scalpel (preferable to scissors).
- Finish with a jet wash.

Wounds that must be left 'open' (no closures/stitches used)

- Animal or human bites
- Puncture wounds
- Penetrating cheek wounds or wounds inside the mouth
- Deep wounds of the hand or foot

- Wounds to joints or tendons
- Wounds over broken bones (open fracture)
- Massive/dirty wounds, wounds with dead or dying tissue inside
- Wounds in the tropics and coral wounds
- Wounds left untreated for more than 8 hours
- Infected wounds

Wounds where it is OK to use closures or stitches
- Clean wounds not involving deeper tissues or organs
- Wounds on the scalp and face
- Delayed closure: after 4 days, a wound that has been left 'open' and is not infected may be closed

Using closures
When closing a wound it is important that no cavities are left below the skin surface, as any such space will fill with fluid, becoming an ideal site for infection. If you cannot eliminate a cavity using deep internal stitches or pressure, leave the wound 'open'. If you do have to close a wound over a cavity, insert a drain (disinfected perforated hydration pack tube) left in the cavity and protruding for 5cm from the lower end of the wound). The drain is gradually removed as healing of the cavity occurs.

Adhesive closures
Steristrips™ are useful and easy to use. Surgical tape is an alternative, as are strips of duct tape or 1cm wide strips of cotton or nylon material with superglue applied. Superglue alone can be used for small wounds (bring the cut surfaces together and smear the glue across the wound, not in it). Don't get superglue on lips or eyelids.

Closures stick best if the skin is dry and hairless, while Benzoin, allowed to become tacky, gives great adhesion for all such closures. Apply one side of the closure to the skin; bring the cut surfaces together with your fingers so they just touch without too much pressure but with no gap between the edges. Then, while pulling on the closure, stick down the other side. Apply the closures 2 to 3mm apart and finish with strips parallel to the wound to stop the closures peeling.

On scalp wounds, long hair can be tied across and fixed with glue or Benzoin.

Stitching (suturing) or stapling

This needs training, a local anaesthetic and knowledge of danger areas where nerves, blood vessels or organs may be damaged by the needle. Cavities in the wound beneath the stitches must be eliminated by correct technique.

Fishing line (disinfected) or cotton can be used as emergency sewing thread.

Removing closures

Leave closures in place for 5 full days for the face, 7 days for the arms and scalp, 10 days for the upper legs, back and hands, up to 14 days for the lower legs and feet. Test the strength of the new scar by removing a closure and gently trying to pull it apart, re-applying the closure if the scar gives way.

Covering (dressing) the wound

Dressing a wound reduces pain, applies some compression to stop bleeding, protects the area and promotes moist wound healing.

Closed wounds

- Cover the wound with a sterile non-stick dressing.
- Bandage the dressing in place.
- Elevate (reduces swelling) and splint lightly (slows spread of infection, prevents wound pulling open).
- Change dressing regularly as described below.

Small open wounds

Just place a non-stick dressing over it (Melolin™, Telfa™, Fixomull™, Opsite™ or clear plastic food wrap such as Clingwrap™, Saranwrap™).

Larger open wounds

These will need moist packing, as this helps stop bleeding, removes debris and absorbs discharges. Large wounds are initially packed tight, while later packing should be looser.

- Place sterile gauze swabs moistened with plain cooled drinkable water in and on the wound (wet the gauze, wring out excess moisture).
- Now add absorbent padding (eg gauze, cotton wool, sanitary pads) and hold in place with a bandage.
- Elevate (reduces swelling) and, if appropriate, splint lightly (slows spread of infection, prevents the wound pulling open).
- Change the packing and the absorbent dressing daily.

Ongoing wound care

If dressings are stuck to the wound, soak them off with warm drinkable water. Take your time (up to 20 minutes) as this can be painful (pain relief may be needed).

- If dressings become wet or dirty, change them immediately (avoid getting it wet – if this is unavoidable, cover dressings with palstic and tape the edges).
- In cooler climates change dressings every two days.
- In the hot tropics change dressings at least twice daily.
- If infection starts, change dressings at least twice daily.
- If the wound is larger than 5cm, start antibiotics.

Complications

Wound infection

Infection is especially aggressive in the tropics and more serious after animal/human bites (particularly to hands and feet) and in open fractures.

As a wound heals there is usually some redness around it, a slight swelling and a little ooze of clear liquid. These normal signs start to settle after two days or so and the wound (or burn) generally feels better each day, often itching in the later stages of healing. If it starts to feel worse, infection is likely. A local infection may spread to the blood stream (septicaemia).

Symptoms and signs

- Pain and swelling, especially if increasing after the first day or two
- Heat (compare with the healthy side)
- Redness increasing around the wound; red streaks may appear and travel up a limb along the lymphatic drainage
- Pus: this may appear as a yellow or green discharge in the wound and often smells bad
- Swelling and tenderness of lymphatic glands central to the wound (groin, armpit or neck)
- Later there may be fever, often spiking (rising and falling) with shivering spells as septicaemia develops

Treatment

- Remove all dressings and remove some or all closures/stitches so that the pus can drain away freely.

- Jet wash the wound 2 to 4 times daily with drinkable water.
- Apply sterile dressings coated in a thin layer of antibiotic ointment. If you don't have an antibiotic ointment, plain white sugar or pure honey is surprisingly effective; apply the sugar/honey paste to the wound, filling all cavities. Then cover with gauze soaked in povi-iodine and dress. When the sugar/honey becomes diluted, jet wash it out and replace it and the dressing. You may have to do this up to 4 times a day.
- Give antibiotics (see Appendix 2) at the very first sign of infection.

Septicaemia

This is a life-threatening infection in the bloodstream. If not treated, death will rapidly occur. It may follow the spread of infection from a wound, splinter, boil or abscess, or from a urinary, kidney, gall bladder or chest infection; or the cause may be unknown.

Symptoms and signs

- Feeling and looking very ill
- Fever with sweating and bouts of shivering chills (rigors)
- There may be red streaks radiating from an infected wound, boil or abscess, with swollen glands
- Agitation, confusion, aggression, delirium and eventually shock

Treatment

Start antibiotics immediately (see Appendix 2).

Tetanus

Tetanus is caused by a bacterial infection and often kills unvaccinated people. Wounds most at risk are puncture wounds, deep or dirty wounds and those with dead tissue in them. The incubation period is usually between 3 days and 3 weeks, but can be much longer.

Symptoms and signs

- Fever, headache, eventually becoming seriously ill
- Increasingly severe muscle spasms, which may cause difficulty swallowing and breathing

Treatment

- Keep the victim calm and still.

- Remove any closures, open the wound and scrub it out as for animal/human bites.
- Give antibiotics (see Appendix 2) and diazepam (5–10mg 6 to 8-hourly) to control spasms.

Specific wounds

Wounds to hands and feet

All but the most superficial injuries to hands and feet are serious. There may be cut tendons, nerves or blood vessels. Infection starts easily, spreads quickly, may be hard to stop and can leave the hand or foot crippled. Fingers or toes may be completely or partially cut off (below). Start antibiotics and evacuate all but minor injuries.

Penetrating object

- **Splinters** may be removed: use a sterile needle to gently dig away enough skin to expose the splinter, and remove it with tweezers. A finger or toe nail may have to be cut away with a scalpel blade to expose a splinter underneath.
- Penetrating objects in the eye, head, abdomen or chest must be left in place unless evacuation is made difficult or impossible by the object.
- Penetrating objects in the hands/arms or feet/legs may be removed if evacuation is delayed for more than 24 hours or there is a problem with splinting, evacuation or pain.
- If an attempt to remove a penetrating object is to be made, do not 'jiggle' the object but try to draw it out smoothly and slowly. Stop if there is strong resistance, a severe increase in pain or a deterioration in CSMS or vital signs. Be prepared for severe bleeding.
- If the object is left in place, apply a ring pad (doughnut bandage) to keep the pressure of dressings off the object.
- Give antibiotics as for wound infection (see Appendix 2).

Fig 14.2 Ring pad (doughnut bandage)

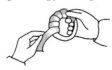
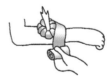

- **Fish hooks** are removed by aligning the shank parallel to the skin surface then, while pressing down on it, use string or pliers to gently extract the barb which is now disengaged. Another method is to push the point onwards out of the skin, then snip off the shank.

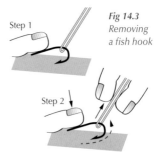

Fig 14.3
Removing a fish hook

Step 1

Step 2

Puncture wounds

These may look insignificant but there is a high risk of infection if there is dirt/foreign objects left inside. Puncture wounds to the abdomen and chest can easily damage internal organs.

- Encourage the wound to bleed freely for a few minutes to flush out any dirt. Then deeply pinch the flesh around the wound, feeling for foreign objects. If you can feel something, use splinter tweezers to try and remove it. You may have to enlarge the entry wound with a scalpel to do this (anaesthetize the wound first). If you suspect there is still some foreign material in the wound, try gently jet washing the wound with drinkable water and/or try compresses of magnesium sulphate paste, sugar paste, honey or molasses, left in place for 12 hours, to bring the foreign material to the surface.
- To prevent infection, keep the wound 'open' (ie without closures). Use tweezers to insert a 'wick' of sterile gauze soaked in antiseptic solution into the wound, replacing it daily as it heals from the bottom up. Place a light dressing over it.

Animal bites

Bites caused by animals (dog, human, monkey, bat etc) are at high risk of becoming infected, especially human bites (which could be a wound on someone's hand from punching someone else in the mouth). Attacks by large animals can cause massive injury due to bites, goring, crushing, trampling or tossing.

- Start antibiotics (see Appendix 2), especially for human bites and animal bites on the hands.
- Unless you can be absolutely sure, assume the animal is a rabies carrier.

Head and neck wounds

Scalp wounds usually bleed heavily but this is easily controlled with pressure (after excluding a fracture) with a suitable dressing. Check for head or spinal injury. Do not apply pressure to neck wounds but carefully pinch the edges of the wound together.

Wounds inside the mouth

Wounds to the tongue, inside the mouth or penetrating the cheek will heal well WITHOUT closures or stitches once the bleeding is controlled. Use a disinfectant gargle 2 or 3 times a day.

See 'Mouth and Teeth' p. 187.

Gaping wounds

- Clean and pack the wound as explained above.
- Tape together any parts that are flopping around approximately into place.
- Add plenty of absorbent dressing and bandage this in place or place a single sheet of plastic on top and secure the edges with adhesive tape and then bandage.
- Change the dressing daily.

Abdominal wounds

If the bowels are protruding from the wound, cover them with a sterile dressing moistened with sterile normal saline solution, add absorbent padding and hold together with broad bandages. Do not push the bowel back into the wound unless evacuation is not possible and the bowel appears to be undamaged. If there is a penetrating wound to the abdominal wall dress it, give nothing by mouth, start recording vital signs and evacuate urgently as organ damage or bowel perforation is likely. If there is any possibility of bowel perforation start antibiotics as for appendicitis (see Appendix 2).

Chest wounds

If a wound has penetrated into the chest cavity, see 'Tension pneumothorax', p. 108.

Gunshot wounds

These high velocity wounds may cause serious internal damage and large exit wounds. The degree of injury depends on luck and the region penetrated.

- Treat as for large open wounds.

Give antibiotics as per wound infection (see Appendix 2) and evacuate urgently for surgical treatment.
See 'Complicated chest injury', p. 108.

Amputation
A limb, digit or part (ear, nose etc) may be cut or torn completely, or partly, from the body during an accident.

Complete amputation
Only undamaged, cleanly severed parts have any chance of being re-attached.
- Clean the amputated part with drinkable water, wrap it in a sterile dressing (or clean cloth) moistened with normal saline solution and place in a plastic bag.
- Cool (but don't freeze) this package by placing on ice or snow, or in cold water. This extends the part's survival time from 4 up to 18 hours (30 hours for fingers). At least cover it with a clean wet cloth to keep cool.

Start antibiotics as for open fracture (see Appendix 2) and evacuate the victim urgently with the amputated part, clearly marked with the time of amputation.

Partial amputation
- If the limb/part/digit is not completely severed, and re-attachment is a possibility, cool the part while evacuating to prolong its survival time and/or to slow the inevitable onset of infection, especially in the hot tropics. Start antibiotics as for open fracture (see Appendix 2).
- If a limb/digit is partially amputated with no CSMS in the end portion and you are more than 24 hours from help, you must consider cutting off the dangling part completely:
  ▶ give painkillers and/or anaesthetize the area and clean the wound
  ▶ apply a tourniquet at the base of a limb/digit just above the damage and complete the amputation with a clean scalpel or scissors
  ▶ cover the wound, apply pressure for at least 10 minutes and elevate to stop bleeding, then slowly release the tourniquet while keeping some compression on the wound. Be prepared to repeat this process.

Crush injuries
When a muscle mass (typically legs or arms) are crushed by a heavy weight, two problems can arise:

121

- **Compartment syndrome:** the compression causes oxygen starvation within the tight internal 'skin' around the muscle mass, resulting in swelling and cell death. It affects just the limb involved, and is very painful.
  - ▸ Remove the crushing object as soon as possible.
  - ▸ Give oxygen, treat shock, check CSMS and evacuate urgently.
- **Crush syndrome:** apart from the possibility of compartment syndrome, the major problem here is the release of toxins from damaged muscles into the victim's circulation. This may cause kidney failure and heart problems, and occurs within one to four hours of the crush event.
  - ▸ Remove the crushing object as soon as possible, but first start giving 1 to 2 litres of liquid (preferably normal saline solution) by mouth, enema or IV.
  - ▸ Give oxygen and start antibiotics as for open fracture (see Appendix 2).

Open fractures

See 'Open fractures' p. 95.

Coral wounds

These are slow to heal, prone to infection and may contain toxins. Pick out any coral fragments with tweezers or a needle, thoroughly clean and keep dry. Treat with antibiotics as for wound infection (see Appendix 2) at the first hint of infection.

Blisters

Blisters are best prevented. Keep feet dry, clean and powdered, use clean dry socks, liner socks and well worn-in footwear.

- At the first sign of chafing (sense of heat) protect the part immediately: change footwear, cover with a blister dressing (eg Moleskin™, duct tape) or adhesive felt (or a thin slice of a closed cell sleeping mat), with a hole to fit the area over the blister.
- Small blisters should be left alone and protected as above.
- If walking is necessary, prick larger blisters with a sterile needle, empty the fluid, leaving the skin in place, clean and protect as above.
- If infection occurs, treat it with antibiotic cream and dressing.

Blood blister under a finger or toenail

This appears as a blue/black area under the nail after a blow. It is not usually a serious injury (although the end bone of the finger may be broken), but can be very painful as the pressure builds up. To release the pain, heat the end of a paperclip over a flame until red-hot and use it to burn a hole in the nail over the centre of the blood blister. No pressure is needed: just rest the hot tip on the nail and after 2 or 3 burns in one spot blood will spurt out, giving instant pain relief.

Nosebleed

Sit the victim up comfortably, leaning forwards. Advise them to spit the blood out, not swallow it. Firmly squeeze the soft part of the nose just below where it joins the bony part, between finger and thumb, for 10 minutes by your watch (20 minutes on hot days or after heavy exercise); repeat as necessary. Place a cold towel/ice pack on neck or forehead.

- If the bleeding continues, smear Vaseline™ on the bleeding area with a cotton bud.
- If bleeding still continues, soak 2 or 3 cotton buds in phenylephrine/ pseudoephedrine nasal drops/spray (or 1:1000 adrenaline solution) and place in the nostril near the front for 5 minutes.
- If bleeding still continues and you have the skills, pack the nose with 60cm of Vaseline-soaked narrow cotton ribbon, or insert and inflate a Foley's catheter or inflate a nasal tampon (eg Rapid Rhino™).
- Do not give aspirin, ibuprofen or similar NSAIDs and stop them if being taken already.
- If the bleeding cannot be stopped, evacuate.

PART 3: Problems and their treatment

15. BITES, STINGS AND NASTY PLANTS

These may cause problems due to trauma, injected venom, allergic reactions or infection. In some cases, there may be breathing difficulties so be prepared to give BLS. If a bite or sting becomes itchy, cover it to prevent scratching, as this is a major cause of infection. See 'Preventing animal and insect bites/stings', p.17.

On land

Snakes

Don't panic! Not all snakes are venomous, not all bites result in injection of venom and venomous snake bites may not lead to death. Do not try to kill or capture the snake.

Symptoms and signs

These vary depending on the species of snake. They can appear in minutes or be delayed several hours. They may include:

- local pain, discoloration and swelling
- bruising and bleeding into tissues
- weakness leading to paralysis; muscle pain
- nausea, vomiting; salivation, sweating
- shortness of breath, difficulty breathing
- visual disturbances; dizziness
- signs of shock, unconsciousness or convulsions.

Treatment for ALL bites

- Keep the victim calm and still
- Check vital signs regularly: be prepared to give BLS
- Do NOT clean the bite site. Do NOT apply a tourniquet or ice/cold compresses, or suction
- Transport to hospital, preferably by carrying or vehicle

In Australia (elapid snakes)

- Apply a PIB (see box below)
- Apply a splint
- If the bite is on body, face or neck apply firm local pressure
- Keep victim still, they should NOT walk

- PIB, SPLINT and IMMOBILITY are the keys to successful first aid

In North America (crotalid snakes)
- Do NOT apply a PIB
- Remove tight clothes or rings as swelling may occur rapidly
- Give pain relief (NOT aspirin or NSAIDs)

Rest of the world
Most bites worldwide occur in rural Africa and India and these bites are usually crotalid, so a PIB is NOT indicated. However if the bite is NOT causing intense local pain and swelling (crotalid symptoms) a PIB may be considered.

PRESSURE IMMOBILIZATION BANDAGE (PIB), PLUS SPLINT

- This lifesaving technique works by slowing or stopping the lymphatic drainage that carries elapid snake venom into the blood circulation. Do not wait for symptoms to appear if an elapid bite is suspected.

  A PIB is also applied to bites from funnel web and black widow spiders, sea snakes, blue ringed octopus and cone shell stings/bites. It may also be applied for ant and bee stings in severely allergic people.

- The bandage and splint are only removed once in hospital.

- Keep the victim as still as possible.

- You will need at least two 10–15cm wide elastic bandages to bind a leg efficiently. Apply the bandages, starting at the bite, going down to fingers or toes then back up to the top of the limb, groin or armpit. They must be tight enough to stop the lymphatic return (you should just be able to slide a finger between bandage and skin) but not so tight that it cuts off the circulation (check CSMS in digits every 30 minutes: if they go white/blue or painful/numb, it is too tight, so loosen and re-apply). A correctly applied bandage feels firm but not painful and may be left in place for hours; it may be applied over trouser legs or shirtsleeves.

- Immobilize the limb with a light splint or put an arm in a sling.

- If the bite is on the body, place a large 10x10cm thick pad of dressing or closed cell mattress over it and firmly bandage in place. You cannot apply a PIB to the neck or head: these bites need URGENT evacuation to hospital.

Spiders

There are thousands of species worldwide: some are harmful but deaths are rare. Fortunately, most bites are minor with just local symptoms.

Common dangerous spiders include brown (or recluse) spider (worldwide), black widow spider (worldwide, warmer climates), funnel web spider (worldwide, especially tropics – a particularly lethal species lives on the east coast of Australia, especially within 200km of Sydney) and red back spider (Australia).

The most dangerous bite location is the face. Bites to small children are more serious than to adults.

Accurate identification of spiders is not easy and quite often the culprit is not seen. What is important is to recognize the onset and progression of symptoms and act accordingly.

Common symptoms and signs

- sharp pain or stinging, and local redness may appear at the bite site. Increasingly serious signs include:
- intense pain or ache gradually increasing in severity. Pain may spread to other locations, including abdomen, chest, neck and head
- local redness turning white as intense blood vessel spasm sets in (which may lead to tissue death). Painful blistering or ulceration at bite site
- swelling and sweating around the bite and/or on the affected limb
- fever, chills, generalized rash and/or sweating
- nausea, vomiting, salivation
- muscle spasm/cramps (especially abdomen and back)
- fits and breathing difficulties
- muscle twitching (including tongue), numbness, tingling lips, weakness
- intense anxiety, confusion, unconsciousness.

Treatment

Treatment is guided by onset of symptoms:
- cover the bite and give pain relief (paracetamol or codeine)
- apply cold compresses to the bite, 20 minutes at a time
- if serious symptoms start to occur, apply a PIB (see box above), give BLS and evacuate urgently
- some antivenoms are available (eg for funnel web spider)
- if the skin ulceration becomes infected, give antibiotics as for wound infection (see Appendix 2).

Bees and wasps

Remove the sting as soon as possible, scrape it off or pick it out. Apply cold compresses and sodium bicarbonate paste. These stings may cause ana-phylactic shock in which case apply a PIB and use the victim's EpiPen™.

Ticks

If undetected, ticks may feed for days or weeks. They may carry nasty dis-eases. Prevention is simple and effective (see Chapter 1, 'Preventing other insect-borne diseases', p. 19). If you find one tick, carry out a thorough whole body search, including belly button, ear canals and all hairy places.

Symptoms and signs

Itching, soreness, redness and swelling around the tick bite. Symptoms and signs of local infection (and often the drainage lymph glands) may appear after a day or two (see 'Wound infection', p. 116). There may be symptoms and signs of the more serious tick infections (see 'Tick-borne diseases', p. 178). Tick bites may cause anaphylactic shock.

Treatment

Most importantly, do not irritate or squeeze the body of the tick, as this will 'inject' saliva, toxins and, possibly, diseases into the victim. Remove the tick with tweezers, preferably fine angled forceps, grasping it as close to the skin as possible, or use thread or dental floss to make a loop round the biting parts close to the skin. If mouthparts are left behind, dig or scrape them out with a disinfected needle. Scrub the bite with disinfect-ant solution. Apply a Band-Aid™ for three days to prevent scratching. Permethrin cream, applied gently to the tick, will kill it but will it still need removal as above.

Mosquitoes, sandflies

Avoid bites (see 'Preventing mosquito-borne diseases', p. 18, and 'Preventing other insect-borne diseases', p. 19). Do not scratch. Treat as for allergy.

Bed bugs, fleas

These bites may cause itchy red lumps, often in groups or lines. Avoid scratching, treat as for allergy. Spread clothing and bedding in the sun, or wash in boiling water.

Leeches
Remove by pulling off. However, if on the eyeball or eyelid, either leave till it falls off or wash with a strong (3%) salt solution (3 teaspoons of salt per litre of water) and apply topical antibiotic eye drops. Control bleeding with a tight Band-Aid™ or small dressing held down firmly with adhesive tape. Leave the Band-Aid™ in place for 4 or 5 days to prevent scratching causing infection.

Scorpions and centipedes
These bites may be venomous or cause severe allergic reactions.

Symptoms and signs
Local burning, pain that may be severe. Salivation, sweating, visual disturbance. Abdominal pain may occur.

Treatment
Apply cold compresses and give painkillers. If the victim starts to feel ill, apply a PIB and splint.

At sea

Sharks and crocodiles
These predators are best avoided (see 'Sharks and crocodiles', p. 17). They can cause massive injury, blood loss and shock. Crocodiles kill by latching on, then rolling their victim, often amputating limbs through the joint as a result.

Jellyfish, barbed fish, sea snakes, cone shells and blue ringed octopus
These marine animals are common and can kill. Unless the animal is clearly seen the cause is not always obvious. The 'Marine envenomation' flowchart in Appendix 7 is a simple aid to working through a complex problem.

General considerations
Jellyfish are found worldwide and their stinging tentacles are responsible for many deaths, especially in tropical and subtropical waters. (**Note:** their numbers and distribution are spreading due to global warning.) They vary widely in size and their tentacles can be many metres long and hard to see. The stings cause pain that may be agonizing, intense, stinging or burning. Skin rashes, irrational behaviour, confusion, disorientation and collapse

may occur. Breathing and circulation may stop very quickly, especially if more than 50% of body surface is involved.

Stonefish, **bullrout**, **scorpionfish**, **zebrafish** and **weeverfish** have poisonous spines on their backs and are sometimes well camouflaged and hard to see. They are found in tropical estuaries, reefs and inlets, but also in temperate waters (eg weeverfish found in southwest England). Extremely severe pain occurs at the site of injury, which spreads up the limb. The skin around the wound may turn grey or blue and the spines may be seen in the wound.

Stingray barbs cause severe burning pain due to venom and trauma, bleeding may be severe.

Sea snakes are found in tropical waters. They are not aggressive or particularly good biters, but their venom is highly toxic. Anxiety, restlessness, dry mouth, nausea, weakness, paralysis and difficulty breathing may occur.

Blue ringed octopus and **cone shell** wounds are usually painless or not severely painful. Numbness of lips and tongue occur with blurred vision, difficulty swallowing and breathing, which may come on rapidly.

General treatment

- get the victim out of the water, reassure and physically restrain them if pain is causing agitation
- follow the flowchart in Appendix 7 'Marine bites and stings'.
- evacuate urgently if the victim shows signs of collapse
- do NOT apply alcohol, methylated spirit, suntan cream, fresh water or urine.

DEACTIVATING VENOM WITH HOT WATER IMMERSION

This means immersion of the affected part in hot water at approximately at 40–45°C, or as hot as you or the victim can comfortably stand it on an uninjured limb) for up to 90 minutes, depending on response.

Alternatives to immersion are: a hot shower; repeatedly pouring hot water; or hot compresses (use a towel or t-shirt) which must be reheated regularly. Even the heat from a candle, lighter or cigar (held some distance from the skin) is effective.

This procedure is lifesaving by preventing pain induced shock and other symptoms. It should be started as soon as possible.

Ciguatera

This is caused by eating fish, caught in tropical or sub tropical waters, which have accumulated certain toxins: it is not uncommon, is temporarily disabling but rarely causes death.

Symptoms and signs

Vomiting, diarrhoea, abdominal cramps; muscle pain, itching, numbness or tingling and clumsiness (ataxia). These may come on within hours or take a couple of days to develop. Symptoms such as headache, tiredness and depression may last for months.

Treatment

Prevent dehydration and treat symptoms. Give ibuprofen for pain relief.

Paralytic shellfish poisoning

Under certain conditions nearly all the shellfish in cooler Pacific waters can occasionally accumulate enough toxin from their diet to cause poisoning.

Symptoms and signs

Numbness of face, arms and legs followed by nausea, headache and loss of coordination, paralysis. Breathing may fail.

Treatment

Get the victim to vomit after drinking two glasses of water.

Scombrotoxic fish poisoning

Poisoning due to breakdown products as certain fish (tuna, mackerel, bonito) decompose. Affected fish have a sharp metallic taste.

Symptoms and signs

Diarrhoea, itching, sweating, rash, headache, vomiting, asthma.

Treatment

Antihistamines, antivomiting medication, avoid doxycycline.

Nasty plants

Worldwide there are plants which can kill you or at least cause pain and disability. Some berries, leaves and mushrooms are highly toxic. Do not eat anything you are not ABSOLUTELY sure about.

Simply touching certain plant species can also be a serious health hazard, especially in the tropics but also in temperate regions. They can cause severe pain, rashes, blisters and leave scars. Some tree leaves have such powerful toxins that even raindrops falling from them can irritate the skin (eg the 'suicide tree'). Other plants can cause blindness through the smoke of burning wood or by rubbing the eyes after touching the leaves.

Avoid contact with all sap, gum, bark or leaves (especially, but not only, hairy ones) of vines, shrubs, trees and cactus unless you know they are safe. Don't swim in algal blooms as some (blue-green algae) can cause skin rashes. Ask for reliable local knowledge.

Some names of nasty plants are: suicide tree, nose burn tree, blinding tree, blister bush, black poison tree and, of course, poison ivy and oak.

The effects may not be immediate and the problem may spread around (eg to the face or eyes) through hands, clothing, tools etc.

Repeated exposure can lead to severe allergic reactions after sensitization.

Treatment
- Specific treatments include washing the area with water, or soapy water for oily leaves.
- Remove spicules very carefully one by one (they break easily leaving the tip in the skin), or use 'depilation strips' eg masking, strapping or duct tape.
- Painkillers, steroids and medical attention may be needed.

See 'Allergy', p. 206, and 'Poisons, bites and stings' in Appendix 10.

PART 3: Problems and their treatment

16. COLD WEATHER PROBLEMS

Prevention is the best approach to the two major cold problems of **hypothermia** (cooling of the body core) and **frostbite** (freezing of an area of skin and tissues underneath). Both problems are common, and they may develop rapidly or slowly. If one person in a group starts to suffer, check everyone else. See 'Safety in extreme climates', p. 20.

Hypothermia

This is when cold causes the temperature of the body's vital internal organs (the 'core' – normally 37°C) to fall. The body's first response to this cooling is to restrict blood flow to extremities. If this response fails to cope, core temperature falls further and shivering starts (shivering is a way of generating heat). With continued core cooling, shivering eventually stops – this is a bad sign.

Once core temperature falls below 35°C, hypothermia is established. If the early stages of hypothermia are promptly recognized, treatment is satisfyingly effective. If core cooling continues, unconsciousness and death occur.

Environmental awareness (cold air, rain, wind, cold water, high altitude) is vital. The air temperature does not have to be below freezing for hypothermia to occur. It may develop quickly (especially with cold water immersion) or more slowly (over several hours). The onset of hypothermia is often missed. Lack of knowledge and lack of prevention (ie inadequate clothing, fitness and food) are major contributing factors. Tiredness and shivering are early signs of hypothermic conditions. Even victims with mild hypothermia may suddenly collapse.

Note: hypothermia, dehydration, low blood sugar (due to not eating), exhaustion and altitude illness (the 'high-altitude quintet' p. 166) share some similar symptoms and signs, so if you find one condition check for the others.

Note: special thermometers are needed to measure core temperature; as this is impracticable in remote situations, symptoms and signs are used to assess the severity of hypothermia, decide on treatment methods and monitor response.

Hypothermia is caused by heat loss through:

- convection: when water or wind passes over the body, carrying heat away (prevented by windproof/waterproof outer clothing)

- conduction: sitting/lying on a surface (or in water) colder than body temperature (prevented by insulation)
- radiation: where the surrounding air is colder than the person (prevented by insulation)
- evaporation: of sweat or water from wet skin or clothing (prevented by dry clothing).

These situations commonly cause hypothermia:
- cold weather with/without rain and/or wind, known as **exposure hypothermia**
- falls into cold water (temperature below 25°C) known as **cold water immersion hypothermia**
- snow avalanches and crevasses.

Other factors promoting hypothermia:
- old people and children are more susceptible
- very high altitude (due to reduction in oxygen)
- trauma (immobility, burns)
- drugs (alcohol, sedatives)
- stroke, lowered level of consciousness
- impaired metabolism, severe infections, malnutrition.

Exposure hypothermia

Symptoms and signs

Early hypothermia
As the victim's core temperature falls towards 35°C they feel cold and may complain about it; their hands and feet will be cold to touch. Shivering may occur as a natural attempt to re-warm.

There may be:
- cold hands and feet, shivering, 'goose bumps' on cold skin (if the victim is shivering, they are *able to stop shivering voluntarily*, even if only for a few seconds)
- tiredness, lethargy, weakness
- poor judgement (denies any problem), irritability, complaining, erratic behaviour.

PART 3: Problems and their treatment

The main point here is that the hypothermic victim who has normal mental function, is still active and talking, will respond well and predictably to immediate treatment.

More severe hypothermia
There may be:
- slurred speech, confusion, irrational behaviour, forgetfulness, apathy
- clumsiness, falling over, muscles become stiff
- violent shivering which cannot be stopped at will (eventually shivering stops)
- lips turn blue and skin is white
- pulse slows with possible heartbeat irregularities
- victim unresponsive, lying down, unconscious, rigid limbs that eventually relax
- breathing and pulse are faint, slow or undetectable – the victim may appear to be dead
- cardiac arrest.

The important point here is that the hypothermic victim who has reduced mental and physical function, or is unconscious, or cannot stop shivering voluntarily (if they are still shivering) will not improve with insulation alone, responding poorly or not at all to attempts to rewarm actively in an exposed environment.

Treatment

Early hypothermia
- Stop and shelter in a safe place, out of the water/wind/rain. Also check and deal with your whole group (see 'Emergency shelters', p. 22).
- Re-warm:
  ‣ If the environment permits, replace wet clothing with dry clothes, add a windproof layer, hat and mittens. If the situation is too exposed to replace wet clothes, add layers over the wet clothes.
  ‣ Speed up re-warming with an insulating Blizzard™ bag/space blanket (a Blizzard™ bag is much better than the original 'space blanket').
  ‣ Put insulation underneath the victim to prevent heat loss to cold ground.
  ‣ Give warm sweet drinks and energy food (sweets, chocolate, sugar, honey).

Once re-warmed and shivering has stopped (due to re-warming), the victim feels better and has no symptoms/signs, they may move on with supervision. Be prepared to stop and repeat the re-warming if symptoms/shivering reappear.

More severe hypothermia
Keep the victim still and lying down flat. Handle them gently as rough handling may stop their heart. Use immobilization techniques (see 'Spinal lift', p. 34) if you have to move them.

- Stop further heat loss. Gently cut off wet clothes, pat (don't rub) their skin dry and gently insert them into a pre-warmed 'hypothermia insulating package'.

HYPOTHERMIA INSULATING PACKAGE

Fig 16.1 Hypothermia insulating package

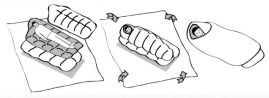

This is an effective means of preventing further heat loss while transporting a hypothermic (or injured victim): lay out your largest waterproof material (canvas, plastic, tarp, sail, tent etc). On this, place several thicknesses of close cell foam mat/inflatable mattress. Add an open sleeping bag and put the victim in a Blizzard bag™ (or space blanket) on top of this. Place another open sleeping bag on all this then fold the lower layers over and secure them, leaving only the face exposed. If the victim is shivering, do not add any external heat; if they are not shivering, add heat by slipping hot water bottles/heat packs/warm rocks into the package, inside (not outside!) the Blizzard bag™/space blanket layer.

- If it is possible to evacuate the victim promptly to expert hospital medical care, do so after insertion into a hypothermia insulating package. If cardiac arrest occurs, start CPR. **Note:** during evacuation, if continuous CPR is not possible, it may be given intermittently (5 minutes CPR, 10 minute pause).

- If evacuation is impossible you will have to organize shelter and attempt active re-warming (this will take many hours):
  - ▸ Place hot water bottles/heat packs (wrapped in a towel or cloth to prevent burns) against their armpits, upper abdomen, neck and groin. Re-heat cooled bottles. Put warm people on either side of the victim while preparing the bottles/heat packs.
  - ▸ Insulate round their face so that the air they breathe is warmed up and/or give assisted breathing.
  - ▸ Warm the tent or room with a stove (beware of CO poisoning).
  - ▸ Give warm sweet drinks/food once able to swallow safely.
  - ▸ The medically trained and equipped may consider giving warm (37 to 41°C) saline solution or saline with dextrose (500ml IV), and oxygen (2–8L/min, ideally pre-warmed).
  - ▸ If the heart stops beating start CPR for 30 minutes.
- If the re-warming is successful, evacuate by stretcher when the victim is conscious, stable and you are sure they won't get cold again during the evacuation process.
- Once in a warm environment, remove any insulation such as Blizzard™ bag/space blanket to allow heat in.

DIAGNOSIS OF DEATH FROM HYPOTHERMIA

- Victim not coming back to life once re-warmed
- Frozen eyeballs (press on them with eyelids closed, compare with a healthy eyeball)
- Frozen chest that cannot be compressed (by chest compressions)
- If medically trained, check for absence of red retinal reflex

Cold water immersion hypothermia

If the victim is likely to be suffering from hypothermia it is vital to get them out of the water while keeping them lying horizontally, as vertical extraction can cause collapse, stopping the heart. Treat as for exposure hypothermia.

See 'In the water', p. 26.

Snow avalanches and crevasses
- Avalanche victims should be given BLS after clearing snow from their airway. Survival rate diminishes rapidly beyond 15 minutes of burial time, but an air pocket and open airway helps survival chances beyond that time. Apply triage if there are several people buried. Make sure searchers are safe.
- In both avalanches and falls into crevasses, assume the victim is suffering from hypothermia and treat. Check for severe injuries.

See Appendix 4.

Frostnip and frostbite

Frostnip and frostbite may occur once the air temperature is near or below freezing. It commonly affects the fingers, toes, face, ears or male genitals; but any surface, exposed or not, is vulnerable. They are more likely to occur at high altitude, in hypothermic or injured victims, if circulation is restricted by tight fitting clothes or boots, with some pre-existing conditions (diabetes, Raynaud's disease) and when taking drugs, such as beta-blockers or nicotine. Prevention is vital as the treatment of frostbite is mainly confined to minimizing the consequences rather than reversing the injury.

Loss of feeling, pain or pins and needles are an early warning that must not be ignored. Frostbite and frostnip are generally not painful till re-warmed (when pain is severe).

Frostnip
This superficial and reversible freezing of a patch of skin is often noticed by the victim's buddy. If not re-warmed, it may progress to frostbite. Frostnip predisposes to frostbite for up to six months.

Symptoms and signs
A patch of skin, sometimes with ice crystals frosting on it, which is white, numb and painless.

Treatment
Re-warm: breathe on the area under cupped hands, press warm fingers on the area. Or place frostnipped fingers or toes in someone's warm armpits, groin or belly. If a return to normal is not accomplished by 10–20 minutes of re-warming, treat as frostbite. Once re-warmed, pain can be severe and last for hours.

PART 3: Problems and their treatment

Frostbite

The skin and some or all of the tissue immediately beneath are frozen, leading to permanent damage. Prevention is vital but skilful first aid will prevent avoidable further damage.

Symptoms and signs

The affected part is white or slightly purple, numb and usually painless. It feels cold, solid or 'woody' to touch and blisters may rapidly appear. A large frostbitten area may eventually turn purple and/or blister.

Treatment

- As soon as safely possible:
  - protect the frozen part from further cold injury (put on dry gloves/mitts/socks) and from trauma. Avoid direct heat from fires or radiators (this can 'cook' the frozen flesh without the victim realizing)
  - treat hypothermia
  - keep the victim warm, hydrated and fed
  - give aspirin 75mg daily and ibuprofen 400mg 8-hourly
  - above 4000m give oxygen (4 to 6L/min)
  - do NOT massage or rub snow on the frostbitten area
  - do NOT smoke or drink alcohol
- Thaw the frostbitten part as soon as possible but only when:
  - there is no danger of re-freezing the newly thawed part, as the 'thaw-refreeze' cycle causes further injury
  - there is no need for the victim to use that part to walk or climb to safety (because once thawed the frozen limb can be cripplingly painful and using it may cause severe damage. This is especially so for the feet and the victim must be carried once frostbitten feet are thawed. Though walking out is OK if only the toes are involved and are well protected).
- Take a series of photos starting before re-warming and seek urgent advice (see Appendix 10 – 'frostbite') as expert treatment can improve outcomes for severe frostbite, especially in the first 24 hours after thawing.
- To thaw the frozen part:
  - Using **active thawing**, the preferred method: suspend the frostbitten part (without touching the bottom or sides) in a large container of warm drinkable water (39 to 41°C, ie as warm as your own hand can comfortably stand for at least half a minute of immersion). Add a dash of betadine. Keep stirring and adding warm water (keep testing with

your hand) during the thawing process, which may take up to one hour. Thawing is complete when the part is un-stiffened, red, throbbing and painful. It may become blistered and swollen. If evacuation is delayed and facilities allow, repeat this re-warming for 30 minutes twice daily.

  ▸ Using **passive thawing** (if you cannot perform active thawing): allow the part to gradually re-warm to the temperature of a warm armpit, abdomen or shelter (hut, tent, sleeping bag etc).

- Elevate the part, air dry, or pat dry. Put sterile dressings between fingers or toes and apply plenty of light padding, remembering that swelling will occur. Do not let the part get cold.
- Strong painkillers may be needed for some weeks (even years) afterwards for severe stinging, burning or electric shock-like pains. Give NSAIDs with added opiates as necessary.
- Any blisters should be left alone unless infected or likely to burst, when they should be drained and dressed.
- If there is traumatic damage or cellulitis/infection appears at the frostbite, give antibiotics as for wound infection (see Appendix 2).
- Check tetanus status.

17. HOT WEATHER PROBLEMS

These are caused by exertion in hot climates, and made more likely by lack of preparation, acclimatization and appropriate clothing. The elderly, children and the less fit are more vulnerable. The most common problem is heat stress, followed by the less common but more serious heat exhaustion and deadly heat stroke. These complaints range from mild to life-threatening. There is always an element of dehydration and salt loss.

Heat stress, heat exhaustion and heat stroke

Heat stress
It is vital to recognize and treat early symptoms of heat stress as it is not painful, easy to ignore and can quickly progress to heat exhaustion or life-threatening heat stroke.

Symptoms and signs
Weakness, dizziness, nausea, feeling faint; may faint briefly.

Treatment
Provide shade, fan them, rest and rehydrate until recovered.

Heat exhaustion
If heat exhaustion is not recognized/treated, heat stroke may develop.

Symptoms and signs
- Tiredness, dizziness, nausea, vomiting, thirst, headache or muscle cramps
- Victim is still sweating and their skin is still elastic
- Temperature is usually normal but may be up to 40°C
- Rapid pulse, low blood pressure (respiratory rate normal)
- Feeling faint or even fainting briefly but with NO reduced level of consciousness before or after a brief faint

Treatment
- Provide shelter from the sun in cool shade with fanning and good ventilation. Insulate from hot ground and rehydrate.
- Lay the victim flat on their back with legs raised if they feel faint, or on their side if they do faint.

- Cool them if their temperature is above normal: fan them while spraying, wiping, sponging or splashing with water.
- Rehydrate (see Chapter 18 'Dehydration' for type and rate of liquid replacement).
- If there is any loss of consciousness (other than brief fainting) or persistent reduced level of consciousness, treat urgently as heat stroke.

Recovery in mild cases of heat exhaustion can be rapid but weakness may persist for days. If the illness is moderate to severe, the victim may be unwell for days and evacuation may be needed.

Heat stroke
This is an emergency. Heat stroke causes death by overheating of the brain and other vital organs. The heat loss mechanisms of the body fail and there is a rapid rise in body temperature. High humidity and exertion are contributing factors. Environmental awareness and early symptoms detection are vital.

Symptoms and signs
Signs and symptoms of heat exhaustion may have been present but now the distinguishing features are:
- persistent reduced level of consciousness or unconsciousness
- there may be sweating or not, with loss of skin elasticity
- raised core temperature (40°C or more)
- fitting and/or shivering may occur
- raised respiratory rate, rapid pulse, low blood pressure.

Treatment
- Evacuate, while cooling the victim aggressively:
  ▸ fan them while spraying, wiping, sponging or splashing with water: the victim may be semi-naked or covered with a wet sheet
  ▸ apply cold wet cloths or ice to the neck, armpits, groin and upper abdomen while continuing to fan and spray the victim
  ▸ if available, use ice cold water, an electric fan or even immerse the victim in cold water
- measuring core temperature rectally is helpful to monitor progress
- give oxygen (6 to 8L/min).

PART 3: Problems and their treatment

Other heat problems

Dilutional (exertional) hyponatraemia (water intoxication)

This dangerously low blood sodium level is much less common than heat stroke It usually occurs in elite athletes in endurance events and requires hospital treatment. In a wilderness setting it is untreatable so prevention is vital. It occurs after long periods of sweating exercise when no food has been eaten but lots of plain water has been drunk. As a result, sodium concentration in the blood drops too low, with little or no dehydration.

Symptoms and signs
- Symptoms are similar to heat stroke.
- Fits are more common than in heat stroke.
- Core temperature may be raised but not as high as heat stroke.
- There is typically no thirst, and urine is still being passed.

Treatment
In a wilderness setting, hyponatraemia is difficult to tell from heat stroke so treat all cases of impaired consciousness as heat stroke (unless able to measure blood sodium level).

Heat edema

Swelling of fingers and ankles may occur in the first few days in a hot environment. It usually settles without treatment.

Prickly heat

This happens when the sweat glands in the groin, under the breasts, around the waist, chest or back get blocked in hot and humid conditions. Itchy areas of redness with spots and blisters appear in the affected areas. If this is widespread, it may predispose to heat exhaustion.

Keep cool, wear loose cotton clothes and avoid scratching. Wash with water only, no soap, and dry the skin. Antihistamines, calamine lotion and/ or hydrocortisone cream help settle itching.

Heat cramps

This is a common problem, solved by gently stretching out and massaging the cramping muscle and drinking salted water.

18. DEHYDRATION

Dehydration means the body lacks sufficient water. Normally water is lost by urinating, sweating and breathing, and amounts to 1.5 to 3 litres per day in normal conditions. Losses may soar to 2 litres per hour or more when exercising in hot, dry conditions.

This water loss may be complicated by accompanying salt loss. When caused by sweating alone, the loss of salts is minimal and is easily replaced by snacking foods. Salt loss becomes significant and must be replaced when the dehydration is caused by vomiting or diarrhoea. Dehydration can progress to shock, unconsciousness and death.

If dehydration is severe or does not improve with treatment, evacuation will be necessary. This is more likely with children and elderly, but even fit young adults may need evacuation. See 'Disinfecting water to make it drinkable', p. 15. Also see 'The high-altitude quintet', p. 166.

HOW TO CHECK HYDRATION STATUS

- A person is **dehydrated** if they pee infrequently, in small amounts that are strong smelling and darker in colour.
- They are **hydrated** if their urine is pale (no darker than champagne colour), frequent, plentiful (at least 1L/day) and doesn't smell.

Thirst is not a reliable indicator of the need to drink (especially at high altitude), as it only appears when dehydration is established, and disappears before one is fully rehydrated: discipline to drink regularly and to check urine frequently is essential.

Causes
- The commonest cause is sweating during exercise especially in hot or dry climates
- Diarrhoea and vomiting
- Less common causes are: burns, severe bleeding, difficulty swallowing and unconsciousness

Symptoms and signs

Early signs
- Tiredness, weakness, lethargy

- Headache, irritability, light-headedness
- Urine is passed infrequently in small amounts, is strong smelling and dark in colour

Later signs
- Clumsiness
- Pale, dry skin with reduced elasticity (tested by skin pinch recoil; compare with a hydrated person)
- Dry mouth and tongue; sunken eyes
- Emotional changes, anxiety, panic, irritability
- Weak rapid pulse and rapid breathing

Treatment
- Identify and treat the cause, and rehydrate.
- Liquids may be given by mouth (see 'Giving liquids by mouth?' p. 67), enema, nasogastric tube or IV, depending on your skill level.
- If treatment is prolonged, monitor the progress:
  ‣ measure and record the vital signs
  ‣ measure and record the volume of all liquid intake (the 'ins')
  ‣ measure the output of urine (have the victim pass urine hourly), and guesstimate the volume of vomit and diarrhoea (the 'outs').
- Now compare the 'ins' and 'outs', making sure the 'ins' are more than the 'outs'.
- Evacuate urgently if dehydration is severe and/or uncontrollable.

Note: liquids given by mouth may cause vomiting, especially if they are salty, sweet or flavoured.

Type of rehydration liquid

Dehydration caused by exercise
- If the victim has been eating regularly, give plain water. This is as good as any sports drink or proprietary rehydration drink.
- If dehydration is severe and not much food has been eaten, give one cup of ORS for every 5 cups of plain water.

Dehydration caused by diarrhoea
Give ORS. Introduce some food after six hours. Children should not be on ORS alone for more than 24 hours.

Dehydration caused by vomiting
Give plain warmish water (or half strength ORS by enema).

Dehydration caused by burns
Give plain water with occasional cups of ORS.

Dehydration caused by external blood loss
Give plain water or normal saline solution (**normal saline solution** is one teaspoon of salt per litre of water).

Dehydration associated with hypothermia
Warm the rehydration liquid (any suitable liquid) to normal body temperature (pleasantly warm to you).

ORS (ORAL REHYDRATION SOLUTION)

This is made up from sachets of premixed salts added to drinkable water, providing sodium chloride (salt), potassium, bicarbonate and glucose.

If no ORS sachets are available, make your own:

- add 8 level teaspoons of sugar and 1 level teaspoon of salt to 1 litre of drinkable water
- to provide potassium (this improves your ORS but is not absolutely essential): add the juice of 1 squeezed lemon (or orange), or 1 cup of coconut water, or half a teaspoon of baking soda; or eat half a mashed banana.

Alternatively:

- give drinks of a solution made up of a 'three finger pinch' of salt plus 2 teaspoons of honey per litre of water, ALTERNATING with drinks of a solution of 1 teaspoon baking soda per litre of water; drink as 250ml alternating 'doses'

    OR

- simpler still, add a fist full of sugar and a three finger pinch of salt per litre of water.

PART 3: Problems and their treatment

How much rehydration liquid should be given?

The amount of rehydration liquid needed to be *given over 24 hours* is worked out from the table below.

MEASURING REHYDRATION NEEDS			
	Mild dehydration	Moderate dehydration	Severe dehydration
BLOOD PRESSURE	normal	dizzy/faint on standing	low blood pressure/shock
HEART RATE	normal	may be raised	raised
EYES	normal	sunken	sunken
SKIN PINCH RECOIL	goes back immediately	goes back slowly	goes back very slowly
MUCOUS MEMBRANES	moist	dry	very dry
CAPILLARY CIRCULATION TEST	< 2 sec	< 3 sec	> 3 sec
THIRST	normal	very thirsty	drinks poorly, unable to drink
URINE OUTPUT	slightly smelly, slightly dark	little output, dark, strong smell	little or no output
Approximate liquid replacement needs over 24 hours *	<50ml per kg of body weight	50-100ml per kg of body weight	100ml per kg of body weight

* To these amounts add the 24-hour normal daily requirement of 25ml per kg of body weight PLUS the guesstimated amount of 'outs' due to diarrhoea, vomiting, blood loss and/or burns.

For example, an 80kg severely dehydrated person will require: 8000ml (100x80) fluid replacement daily + 2000ml (25x80) normal daily requirement = 10,000ml (10 litres) + any guesstimated amount of 'outs', over 24 hours.

Rate of rehydration

The rate depends on the severity of the problem and the way by which the liquid is given. Adults can only absorb so much liquid by mouth at a time without vomiting, so give no more than a maximum of 200ml every 15 minutes.

- Approximate rates for an adult:
  ▸ by mouth: start with sips, building up to 200ml every 15 minutes; give half the total volume required in the first 8 hours and the rest over the next 16 hours
  ▸ by enema: do not exceed 200ml/hour
  ▸ by nasogastric tube: do not exceed 200ml/hour as this may provoke vomiting/inhalation
  ▸ by IV: larger volumes can be given at a faster rate
- Tail off to a maintenance amount of liquid once vital signs are coming back to normal and the victim is feeling better and eating. Satisfactory hydration is achieved when over one litre of pale/non-smelling urine is passed every 24 hours.

19. DIARRHOEA AND FOOD POISONING

Diarrhoea is a soft or watery bowel motion with an increase in frequency. The two commonest causes of diarrhoea in travellers are an infection due to germs (viruses, bacteria or protozoa) or a change of diet. The infection invades by drinking or eating contaminated water or food, or by touching contaminated objects (eg hands, door handles, prayer wheels etc).

Food poisoning is the abrupt onset of vomiting (with or without diarrhoea but vomiting predominates) caused by eating food contaminated by toxin-producing bacteria.

See 'Preventing diarrhoea and food poisoning' p. 14, and Chapter 20, 'Abdominal (belly) problems'.

Mild diarrhoea

This is usually caused by a change of diet or a virus. In either case, an antibiotic will not help and might make things worse.

Symptoms and signs
- Less than 3 or 4 loose/watery bowel motions within 24 hours
- Eating usually makes the symptoms worse and some colicky abdominal pain may occur
- Symptoms will eventually disappear over 2 or 3 days with no antibiotic treatment.

General treatment
- If there are no symptoms of dehydration and the victim is still eating, plain water is sufficient. If symptoms and signs of dehydration appear, give ORS alone.
- Avoid foods and drinks that make symptoms worse (eg alcohol, coffee, chillies, fatty/high energy food). Choose a bland diet (eg boiled rice, porridge, plain biscuits); it is not necessary to limit the quantity of food unless it makes the symptoms worse.
- Anti-motility drugs, eg loperamide (Imodium™), Lomotil™ or codeine may be given to slow the frequency of bowel motions, reduce abdominal pain, control dehydration or while travelling. **Note:** anti-motility drugs do not treat the underlying infection. When using them, avoid constipation: aim to give just enough to control excessive frequency, pain and dehydration.

Severe diarrhoea

Severe diarrhoea in developing countries is usually due to bacteria or protozoa (giardia, amoeba). It will often need antibiotic treatment (90% of diarrhoea cases in travellers seen by doctors in Nepal need antibiotics), especially if the diarrhoea persists or dehydration cannot be controlled.

Symptoms and signs
- More than 4 loose/watery bowel motions within 24 hours, PLUS one or more of the following symptoms:
  - ▶ fever, nausea, vomiting, stomach cramps
  - ▶ mucus or blood may appear in the stools
  - ▶ victim feels and looks ill
  - ▶ victim is becoming dehydrated.

Treatment
General treatment above, plus:
- Give antibiotics: try to decide on the cause of the diarrhoea using the descriptions below and Fig 19.1. See Appendix 2 for the appropriate antibiotic.
- If the cause of the diarrhoea cannot be decided, follow the 'Antibiotic protocol for severe diarrhoea of unknown cause' (p. 151).
- If vomiting persists, treat it.
- If the diarrhoea (or vomiting) does not improve with treatment, and especially if dehydration cannot be controlled, evacuate.

Bacterial diarrhoea
This is the commonest cause of severe diarrhoea in developing countries and is approximately 10 times more frequent than giardia. It may last one to two weeks or more.

Symptoms and signs
- Rapid onset with the victim usually feeling ill. Symptoms appear 24 to 48 hours after infection and, over days, may spread through a group due to poor hygiene.
- Frequent loose/watery bowel motions (more than 4 within 24 hours)
- Fever, nausea, vomiting, stomach cramps
- Possible blood and/or mucus in the stools

PART 3: Problems and their treatment

Giardia

Giardia is a protozoa that causes longer lasting diarrhoea (weeks or months). Symptoms may eventually settle without treatment and the victim may become a carrier.

Symptoms and signs

Symptoms develop at least one week after the initial infection and possibly up to 3 weeks later. They usually develop slowly over some days (but in a few cases can start suddenly and explosively along with fever).

- Diarrhoea frequency and symptoms may be mild or severe.
- Bowel motions can be loose, gassy and explosive. There may be the classic bad-egg-smell burps or farts (but note these may also happen in bacterial diarrhoea).
- Victim may experience stomach cramps or pain soon after eating.
- They may suffer increasing fatigue and weight loss over weeks or months.

Amoebic diarrhoea

Amoebae are protozoa found worldwide, especially in the tropics. Amoebic diarrhoea is uncommon in travellers. It is hard to distinguish from giardia but is less common and more serious.

Symptoms and signs

- Diarrhoea developing slowly over a period of days
- Porridge-like, smelly stools sometimes containing blood and/or mucus
- Cramps or abdominal pains especially while passing a motion
- Fever, nausea or vomiting
- If not treated, may last months and produce extreme fatigue and weight loss

Cyclospora

This blue-green alga is common in monsoon seasons. There is sudden onset of diarrhoea (watery bowel motions that can last for weeks), often with fever, nausea or vomiting, followed by loss of weight and appetite.

Cryptosporidum

'Crypto' is a waterborne protozoal disease causing stomach cramps, fever, nausea or vomiting. It may cause weight loss, but in a healthy person it usually settles after a couple of weeks. Antibiotics don't work well.

Typhoid

Typhoid may be a cause of diarrhoea. See p. 179.

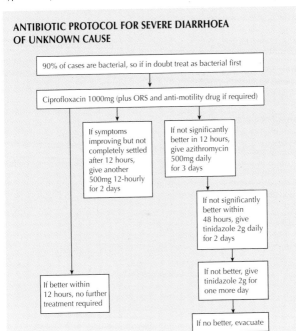

ANTIBIOTIC PROTOCOL FOR SEVERE DIARRHOEA OF UNKNOWN CAUSE

90% of cases are bacterial, so if in doubt treat as bacterial first

Ciprofloxacin 1000mg (plus ORS and anti-motility drug if required)

If symptoms improving but not completely settled after 12 hours, give another 500mg 12-hourly for 2 days

If not significantly better in 12 hours, give azithromycin 500mg daily for 3 days

If not significantly better within 48 hours, give tinidazole 2g daily for 2 days

If not better, give tinidazole 2g for one more day

If better within 12 hours, no further treatment required

If no better, evacuate

Persistent diarrhoea

When diarrhoea does not improve despite treatment, there are several possible reasons.

- The infecting germ may be resistant to the antibiotic you have given or the course of treatment was not long enough.
- The diarrhoea may be caused by a virus or other germ that does not respond to antibiotics.
- Antibiotics themselves (especially repeated courses) may be the cause of persistent diarrhoea.

- There are several non-infective causes of persistent diarrhoea, some of which are serious medical conditions such as tropical sprue, colitis.

If the diarrhoea returns once you are home or if any symptom persists, see a doctor for investigation and diagnosis.

Food poisoning

This is caused by eating food contaminated by toxin-producing bacteria. The onset of symptoms is within hours of ingestion. It may affect several people eating the same meal, or just one person.

Symptoms and signs
The onset of symptoms is typically sudden and often violent.
- Nausea and vomiting which can be severe
- Abdominal cramps
- Victim pale, sweating; looking and feeling unwell
- Possible diarrhoea accompanying or following the vomiting

The victim is usually better (or improving rapidly) in 12 to 24 hours.

Treatment
- Treat vomiting and rehydrate.
- If the victim continues to vomit and is becoming weak and dehydrated, evacuate.
- No antibiotics are needed unless severe diarrhoea develops.

Fig 19.1 Diagnostic aid to non-viral diarrhoea in developing countries

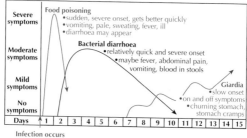

20. ABDOMINAL (BELLY) PROBLEMS

The abdomen (belly) contains the stomach, intestines, liver, gallbladder, pancreas, spleen, kidneys, bladder and the internal female and male organs. The spinal column and major blood vessels are at the back, and there is a thin layer of muscles in front. Chest problems and women's/men's problems can cause abdominal pain.

The common problems are easily recognized and dealt with but it is often difficult or impossible to decide on the cause when a serious problem develops. However, you can draw general conclusions and arrive at the appropriate treatment by carrying out a thorough secondary survey with vital signs. Treat the symptoms and be ready to evacuate if pain persists or the victim's condition worsens.

Common abdominal problems

Constipation

This is caused by dehydration, diet change and some medications (eg codeine, loperamide). It can be acute or chronic, with discomfort and bloating.

Treatment

- Treat it as soon as possible: increase fibre in the diet (eg cereals, fruits), drink plenty of liquid, especially hot drinks (coffee) first thing in the morning.
- Give 1 or 2 laxative tablets at night; as a last resort, use an enema of (cool) black coffee.

Indigestion and heartburn

Symptoms and signs

- Sharp or burning pains in the upper abdomen (**indigestion**)
- Acidity, sourness or burning rising to the back of the throat, with or without mouth-watering (**heartburn**) which may wake the victim in the night
- Symptoms either improved or made worse by eating.

Treatment

- Eat small snacks every 2 to 4 hours (if this does not make symptoms worse); try sleeping half sitting up or with the head of the bed raised.
- Chew antacid tablets, 2 to 8 tabs a day.
- Take ranitidine (150mg 12-hourly) if not improving.

- Avoid tobacco, carbonated drinks, alcohol, high calorie or fatty foods.
- Avoid aspirin, ibuprofen and other NSAIDs.

Nausea and vomiting

Nausea and vomiting are common problems, with many causes including: food poisoning/bacterial diarrhoea, sea/motion sickness, heart attack, head injury, meningitis, malaria, irritation of the inner ear by a virus (**viral labyrinthitis:** nausea/vomiting, dizziness, 'spinning', vertigo) and serious abdominal problems (described below). Other causes include allergy/intolerance to medications especially penicillin, erythromycin, codeine and NSAIDs.

General treatment of vomiting

Carry out a secondary survey, try to work out the diagnosis and follow the treatments suggested. If vomiting continues and there are no contra-indications:

- Once the victim is 'retching' (when the stomach is empty after 3 or 4 good vomits and the victim is bringing hardly anything up), give half a glass of warm water to sip and 1 or 2 antacid tablets to chew.
- If vomiting/retching continues and is causing problems such as dehydration or exhaustion, and if medical help is unavailable, give antivomiting medication:
  - by mouth (prochlorperazine/Stemetil™): crush the tablets and give with sips of water; this is likely to be effectively absorbed if the victim can hold it down for 30 minutes before vomiting again. If vomiting occurs within 10 minutes of giving the medication, repeat the dose once
  - buccal (prochlorperazine/Buccastem™): place on the gum behind upper lip
  - sublingual (ondansetron/Zofran Zydil™ wafers): allowed to dissolve on tongue
  - suppository (prochlorperazine/Stemetil™, or promethazine/Phenargan™)
  - IM injection (prochlorperazine/Stemetil™) if trained
  - enema (see p. 36).
- Rehydrate: encourage frequent tiny sips (not large gulps) of plain warmish water and continue even if vomiting persists, as water is rapidly absorbed from the stomach; consider an enema if dehydration occurs.
- If vomiting persists, becomes projectile or if there is blood or faeces in it, or the victim is becoming dehydrated, weak or ill, treat as a serious abdominal problem and evacuate.

Serious abdominal problems

There are many serious causes of abdominal problems. In addition, there are several conditions outside the abdomen wich may present with abdominal symptoms (usually pain and/or tenderness); these include pneumonia, pelvic injury, heart attack and some problems specific to women or men (see appropriate chapters).

Common symptoms and signs

Serious problems often start with only mild symptoms. You may not find the exact diagnosis, but what is important is early recognition of serious signs and symptoms and any progressive worsening.

Pain may be constant (injury, ulcer, gallbladder infection, pneumonia, heart attack) or may come and go as spasms/cramps/colic (kidney stones, bowel obstruction) or a combination of both (hernia) at different times:

- they may be lying down, crouched over, clutching their belly and in distress
- increasing tenderness or pain when pressing (with flat of fingers) on the abdomen
- increasing stiffness/rigidity of the abdominal muscles
- swelling of abdomen or a mass felt under the abdominal muscles, or in the groin (hernia)
- diarrhoea or constipation
- vomiting, which may be:
  ▸ projectile (vomit is forcefully spewed)
  ▸ containing blood (fresh red or looking like coffee grounds)
  ▸ smelling like faeces
  ▸ persistent.
- blood from the anus (back passage), either fresh (see 'Haemorrhoids', p. 203), fresh blood mixed with stools, or black, older blood passed as black tarry stools that smell awful
- signs of shock.

General management

- Put the victim in the most comfortable position (eg half sitting, crouching, curled up).
- Monitor and record vital signs, and regularly repeat your examination of the abdomen (gently, fingers flat on the skin, avoiding jabbing or poking).
- Nothing by mouth if evacuation is possible within 6 hours, otherwise see 'Giving liquids by mouth?', p. 67.

155

- If evacuation is delayed and vomiting is causing dehydration/exhaustion, treat the vomiting.
- Evacuate urgently if there are any of the following:
  - ▶ pain in abdomen after forceful injury
  - ▶ severe pain lasting more than 6 hours
  - ▶ persistent (not wave-like) constant pain lasting 12–24 hours
  - ▶ vomiting blood or vomit smells of faeces
  - ▶ blood from the anus (black, tarry, sticky, smelly stools or the persistent passage of copious amounts of fresh blood) without an obvious bleeding haemorrhoid
  - ▶ blood in the urine after an abdominal injury
  - ▶ dehydration cannot be controlled
  - ▶ persistence/worsening of any of the common signs and symptoms mentioned above.

Specific serious abdominal problems

Acute ulcer of the stomach (peptic ulcer)

Symptoms and signs
- Severe upper abdominal pain before or after meals, or pain waking the victim up in the night
- Constant burning pain in the upper abdomen, which may be felt in the back
- Pain that is relieved for a short time by antacid tablets
- Vomiting blood or passing blood in stools (which will be black, tar-like and smell awful) – this is a serious sign

Treatment
Treat as for indigestion, especially with ranitidine, and see 'General management' above.

Appendicitis

Symptoms and signs
- Typically, mild to moderate pain in the centre of the abdomen that shifts after a few hours to the lower right-hand side of the abdomen and becomes more severe. Pain is made worse by movement and coughing. The lower abdomen, especially on the right, becomes tender to touch

- The abdominal muscles become increasingly rigid as the appendicitis progresses
- Possibly vomiting, loss of appetite, mild diarrhoea, a low fever and an increased pulse rate
- The symptoms of appendicitis usually become severe within 48 hours of onset. Without treatment, it does one of three things: gets better, forms an abscess or develops into **peritonitis** (a general inflammation/infection of the abdomen leading to shock and death). See also 'Pelvic infection' p. 195.

Treatment

If you think the person may be suffering from appendicitis:
- Evacuate immediately (best to carry them).
- If evacuation is not available or will be delayed, start the following treatment:
  ‣ rest, sips of plain water and occasional cups of ORS; no food
  ‣ give antivomiting medication to control persistent vomiting and prevent dehydration; give painkillers (paracetamol or codeine) if pain is severe. Do not give laxatives
  ‣ give antibiotics (Appendix 2). This non-surgical treatment of appendicitis is surprisingly effective and can also be used for acute infection of the gallbladder.

Bladder obstruction

See 'Pelvis' p. 107.

Bowel obstruction

This is more common in people with a previous history of abdominal surgery, when the bowel becomes twisted around an old internal scar. A hernia may cause obstruction.

Symptoms and signs

- A pain in the abdomen that comes and goes (**colic**)
- Swelling and tenderness of the abdomen that follows the pain
- Constipation and/or vomiting which may become projectile
- Breath or vomit smelling like faeces

Treatment

See 'General management', above. Give nothing by mouth. Evacuate urgently.

PART 3: Problems and their treatment

Hernia

This is a protrusion of bowel through a torn muscle (but still under the skin), usually due to heavy lifting/straining, which commonly occurs in the lower abdomen/groin, or around the belly button.

Symptoms and signs

- A bulge appears when standing, coughing or straining. The victim may report a tearing sensation or pain when this first happens. There may be a dragging or aching pain, or no pain at all.
- The bulge often disappears spontaneously ('reduces') on lying down, only to reappear when standing again.

Treatment

- If there is no pain and the bulge reduces easily, the victim may decide to continue their trip.
- If pain develops and the bulge becomes stuck (irreducible, especially likely in the upper thigh) and tender, evacuate urgently for surgery. Treat as for appendicitis.

Gallstones

Gallstones may cause problems in the gallbladder and its drainage tube.

Symptoms and signs

- Severe pain, intermittent (colic) or constant, in the right upper part of the abdomen
- Possible pain at the right shoulder tip or the back of the lower chest
- Pain on pressing under the right hand side ribs as they take a deep breath
- Nausea and vomiting
- Eyes or skin turning yellow (jaundice) due to a stone blocking bile drainage. **Note:** if jaundice is present, try to avoid medications: if you must give them, use half the usual dose. See 'Hepatitis A', p. 180

Treatment

- If evacuation is delayed, give plain water and occasional cups of ORS, but no food.
- Give painkillers: ibuprofen or naproxen (add codeine if needed), OR diclofenac suppositories 50mg 12-hourly (do NOT use this suppository with any other NSAID eg ibuprofen, diclofenac etc).

- Give antivomiting medication to control persistent vomiting and prevent dehydration.

Acute infection of the gallbladder

This is similar to gallstones but the pain is constant and fever is present. Follow the same guidelines and treatment as for appendicitis, plus pain relief as for gallstones.

Kidney stones

Stones may cause problems in the kidneys or bladder, or their drainage tubes. See also 'Kidney infection' p. 194.

Symptoms and signs

- Sudden onset of pain in the mid-lower back on one side, or in the lower abdomen (bladder) which may extend down into the genitals
- Pain usually severe and typically intermittent (colic) although it may be constant
- Nausea or vomiting
- Desire to pass urine (caused by stones in the bladder)
- Blood in urine

Treatment

- Give 4 litres of liquid to drink every 24 hours to help flush out the stones.
- Give painkillers (diclofenac suppository 50mg 8 or 12-hourly OR ibuprofen or naproxen. Add paracetamol or codeine if needed).

Internal bleeding into abdomen

This may be due to injury or disease.

Symptoms and signs

- Injury, pain or tenderness of the abdomen
- Vomiting blood. **Note:** if one cup of blood has been vomited, two more cups are likely to be going down the intestines
- Passing blood from the vagina, penis or anus (colour and consistency may vary from bright red blood to dark black tarry stools)
- Symptoms and signs of shock

Treatment

See 'General management' above and evacuate.

21. RESPIRATORY PROBLEMS

Respiratory tract infections include simple head cold, flu (influenza), throat
infection, tonsillitis, laryngitis, glandular fever, sinusitis, middle ear infections, bronchitis, tracheitis, pleurisy and pneumonia. Infections may be viral
or bacterial and spread by cough, sneeze or contact with infected surfaces.

Non-infective respiratory problems include asthma, CO poisoning, high
altitude dry cough, HAPE, problems caused by diving, spontaneous pneumothorax and pulmonary embolus.

Once a diagnosis is made, refer to the appropriate section in this book.

Respiratory tract infections

It is often impossible to know exactly what the problem is. A simple cold
may progress to something more serious, such as bronchitis. Rapid worsening is a serious sign.

A repeated secondary survey, observation of the victim and vital signs
will help decide the severity of the problem and how to treat. Fevers should
be measured by thermometer.

Symptoms and signs

- Blocked runny nose, sneezing and/or feeling unwell (**head cold**)
- Sore throat (look at the back of the victim's throat and tonsils with a good
  light, gently holding their tongue down with a clean spoon handle). There
  may be redness in the throat (**throat infection**). The tonsils might be bright
  red, with or without pus as tiny white/yellow blobs (**tonsillitis**)
- The victim's voice sounds hoarse and they have difficulty talking, or lose
  their voice altogether (**laryngitis**). This is usually a viral infection and
  antibiotics are not needed
- These last three complaints may cause pain/difficulty swallowing, talking or coughing
- Headache with stuffiness, pain and tenderness around the eyes and
  nose, worse for hanging the head down, possible pus dripping from the
  nose or down the back of the throat (**sinusitis**)
- Shivering, muscle aches and fever (**influenza – 'the 'flu'**)
- Cough (check whether they suffer from asthma; if at altitude, could it be
  HAPE?). There may be green/yellow sputum, especially in the morning
  (**bronchitis**). A sudden onset of cough, shortness of breath, pain on breathing or coughing with high fever may be a sign of life-threatening **pneumonia**

- Sharp, localized chest pain on breathing or coughing (**pleurisy**)
- Enlarged tender glands in the neck (**glandular fever**)
- Pain in the central chest, especially on coughing (**tracheitis, bronchitis**)
- Tiredness and depression may persist for weeks, particularly after glandular fever or flu

General treatment

Rest. Keep well hydrated. Avoid foods which encourage and thicken mucus production (eg dairy products). Wear a scarf across mouth and nose in cold, dry or dusty conditions. Depending on the symptoms, give any of the following:

- **Sore throats:** Suck on medicated throat lozenges (eg Strepsils™). Gargle for sore throat: gargle (but do not swallow) warm salted water or an aspirin solution (2 tabs in a glass of warm water) 2 to 4-hourly.
- **Blocked nose:**
  ‣ Nasal washout: gently sniff and spit out a warm normal saline solution from a cup, into one nostril at a time while blocking the other one, 8 to 12-hourly.
  ‣ Steam inhalations: inhale steam from a bowl, pot or cup of hot water for 5–10 minutes several times a day. Place a towel over the head and add tincture of benzoin, tiger balm or eucalyptus oil for extra effect.
  ‣ Nasal decongestant drops or spray are usually effective: 1 spray, or 3–4 drops, in each nostril with the head hanging upside down, or lying down head tilted right back, 6 to 8-hourly or just at night, for a maximum of 5 days.
  ‣ As appropriate, give sinus and flu tablets.
- **Headache, flu-like pains:** give painkillers (paracetamol, aspirin or ibuprofen).
- **Wheezy breathing** or if chest feels 'tight', use an asthma reliever spray.
- **Chest filled with mucus:** postural drainage of sputum: encourage/help the victim to cough up sputum by patting them vigorously on the back while lying down with head lower than the feet, positioning them on their side, back, then front.
- **Difficulty breathing:** Give oxygen (6 to 8L/min).
- Antibiotic treatment may be necessary (see specific problem in Appendix 2), especially if the victim has asthma or emphysema, or in these situations:
  ‣ **tonsillitis** or **severe throat infection** with worsening swallowing problems

- ‣ **sinusitis** with temperature above 38.0, severe symptoms or not settling after 7 days
- ‣ **bronchitis** where the victim is unwell, has a fever, is short of breath or if the infection is not improving after 4 days
- ‣ if **pneumonia** or **pleurisy** is suspected and the victim is ill.
- If **glandular fever** is suspected (mainly in teenagers/young adults – slow onset of sore throat, very swollen neck glands, muscle aches), antibiotics have no effect. Avoid contact sports or activities where there is a risk of a blow to the abdomen, as the spleen may rupture.
- Evacuate if infection gets worse, with fever or shivers, or if it interferes with breathing.

Non-infective respiratory problems

Asthma

Asthmatics usually carry their regular medications but in a wild setting should also carry (and know how to use) a short-acting asthma reliever spray (eg salbutamol), a spacer (Fig 21.1), a 2-week course of prednisolone tablets and, in case of a chest infection, antibiotics as for bronchitis (see Appendix 2).

Asthmatics often feel well at altitude, but episodes may be triggered by respiratory tract infections, exercise, cold and/or dry air, dust, pollen, animal hair, food allergy or stressful situations.

Symptoms and signs

Attacks range from mild to severe.

Mild attack: annoying cough, especially at night, mild difficulty breathing, mild wheeze.

Severe attack: distress, confusion, fighting for breath; respiratory rate either increased (over 25 breaths/min) or decreased (under 8 breaths/min – this is a very serious sign), tiring rapidly, speaking only in short bursts of a few words at a time, wheeze may be absent and the chest ominously silent. Unconsciousness may follow.

Treatment

- Stop, rest and reassure. Sit the victim up with arms on a support in front of them (eg on a table) in a warm, humid environment and encourage them to relax. Ask what their emergency action plan is. Check they are using their asthma spray correctly.
- Give oxygen for a severe attack.

- Stop aspirin, ibuprofen and any other NSAIDs.
- Use their *reliever* asthma spray (blue or grey coloured eg salbutamol) with a spacer (see below) as follows:
  - ▸ 4 puffs (each separated by 4 breaths), re-assess grade for 4 minutes. If no improvement:
  - ▸ 4 puffs (each separated by 4 breaths), re-assess grade for 4 minutes. If no improvement:
  - ▸ 10 puffs (each separated by 4 breaths), re-assess grade for 20 minutes. If no improvement:
  - ▸ continue with 10 puffs every 20 minutes until improvement occurs.
- If improvement occurs at any point in the above protocol, give ongoing treatment as follows:
  - ▸ mild attack: 4 puffs every hour
  - ▸ moderate attack: 10 puffs every hour
  - ▸ severe attack: 10 puffs every 20 minutes.
- Continue the victim's usual asthma *preventer* spray (yellow, beige or brown coloured) but double their usual dose.
- Treat any throat or chest infection.
- At altitude, check for HAPE and treat for both if it cannot be excluded.
- Seek medical help/evacuate urgently if:
  - ▸ the original attack was severe, or
  - ▸ the attack is not controlled by the above protocol after 2 hours, or
  - ▸ symptoms return within 2 hours of a successful treatment.
- If medical help/evacuation is not available and the attack is moderate or severe: give prednisolone (40mg at once, and then 40mg each morning

USING A SPACER

A spacer device greatly improves the action of asthma sprays. To make one, cut a hole in the side of a plastic bottle (up to a 1-litre size) to loosely fit round the spray's mouthpiece (but do not seal round it, as enough air must be allowed in for a deep breath).

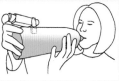

Fig 21.1 Spacer

The victim puts the neck of the bottle in their mouth, activates the spray once and takes four deep breaths of the now invisible vapour (this is the equivalent of one 'puff' in the treatment outlined).

until symptoms improve – usually 5 days – then 10mg daily until medical advice is available). Prednisolone takes 4 hours to work. **Note:** dexamethasone is a substitute for prednisolone, the dose is the same as for HACE, but the duration is as described here for prednisolone.

HAPE

HAPE (high altitude pulmonary edema) has symptoms similar to other respiratory problems. Occasionally HAPE may result in infection and look like pneumonia. HAPE is much more common than pneumonia at altitude. If in doubt, treat for both and descend (see 'HAPE', p. 168).

High altitude dry cough

The cold dry air of high altitude may cause a chronic, dry, persistent cough. There is no infection, no fever, no increased respiratory rate, no chest signs and no loss of performance. Check regularly for HAPE and asthma. Antibiotics are useless. If the cough is severe and causing distress, descend.

Carbon monoxide (CO) poisoning

CO is a colourless odourless gas produced by combustion. Poisoning occurs when cookers, open flames, gas heaters and internal combustion engines are used in confined spaces such as tents, snow holes, vehicles in snowdrifts or boats with inadequate ventilation. There may be no warning at all and unconsciousness and death may quickly follow.

Symptoms and signs
- Possible mental changes, with the victim not wanting to admit there is anything wrong
- Headache, nausea, shortness of breath, panting, chest pain
- Fainting, drowsiness, unconsciousness

Treatment
- Don't become a victim while attempting a rescue: use a damp cloth as a temporary mask.
- Move the victim outside or into another shelter; keep them quiet.
- Give oxygen (10 to 15L/min). If oxygen is not available, treat in a hyperbaric bag for several hours, or give assisted breathing.

Pneumothorax
See 'Chest injuries' p. 108.

22. ALTITUDE ILLNESS – AMS, HACE AND HAPE

Altitude illness becomes common above 3000m and presents in the following ways:

- AMS (acute mountain sickness): very common but not life-threatening unless ignored
- HACE (high altitude cerebral edema): common and life-threatening
- HAPE (high altitude pulmonary edema): common and life-threatening (more common above 4000m).

AMS incidence ranges from 20–80% of people going to altitude (the higher one goes, the more frequent the AMS). HAPE is roughly twice as common as HACE, and together they occur in approximately 1–2% of people going to high altitude. These three forms of altitude illness can vary from mild to severe, and may develop rapidly (over hours) or slowly (over days). AMS may progress onto HACE, while HACE and HAPE can occur individually or together.

Warning: people often refuse to admit they have altitude illness and blame their symptoms on cold, heat, infection, alcohol, insomnia, exercise, unfitness or migraine. Continuing to ascend when symptoms and signs of altitude illness are present, however mild, has led to many deaths.

The Golden Rule: if you are unwell at altitude and getting worse, DESCEND!

See 'At high altitude' p. 23.

Acclimatization

As you ascend above 2500m, your body acclimatizes to the decreasing amount of oxygen available. At 5500m there is only half the oxygen in each breath. Effective acclimatization to any given altitude takes a week or so, but full acclimatization takes six weeks.

As one acclimatizes to higher altitude, breathing speeds up and become deeper, more urine is passed and blood slowly thickens with extra red cells. If ascent is too fast and/or the height gain too much, these mechanisms of acclimatization do not have time to work, and symptoms and signs of altitude illness (also called high altitude illness or altitude sickness) appear.

If the victim has mild symptoms and signs of AMS and rests at the same altitude, symptoms usually disappear over several hours (but in some people this can take up to 3 days!) and they are now acclimatized to this altitude. AMS may reappear as they ascend higher, as acclimatization to the new altitude has to take place all over again. If AMS symptoms are severe, descent is necessary: this will settle the problem and re-ascent can then be undertaken.

Individuals vary between 'fast' and 'slow' acclimatizers and need different ascent rates. A flexible schedule is best as it allows rest days. The reality is that many trekkers are on tight schedules (especially so on some commercial treks) and this leads to a higher incidence of altitude illness. However, factors such as pride, peer pressure, rivalry and ignorance can lead trekkers on flexible schedules to ascend too quickly. Slow acclimatizers on tight schedules are at extra risk: identify them as soon as possible.

	Flexible schedule	Tight schedule
Fast acclimatizers	LOWER RISK	MEDIUM RISK
Slow acclimatizers	MEDIUM RISK	HIGH RISK

PERIODIC BREATHING

When sleeping at altitude, most people suffer from periodic breathing to some degree. It is recognized by repeated cycles of normal or fast breathing followed by breath holding, then several gasping breaths. The sufferer often wakes feeling like they are suffocating. This can be frightening for the sufferer's tent 'buddy'. In the morning the victim often feels tired and unwell.

Periodic breathing does not appear to precipitate HACE or HAPE.

Treatment: acetazolamide, the 'high-altitude sleeping pill', 125–250mg two hours before sleep.

THE HIGH ALTITUDE QUINTET

Altitude illness, **hypothermia**, **dehydration**, **low blood sugar** (due to not eating) and **exhaustion** all share similar symptoms and signs and can occur together.

If any of these symptoms and signs are present, check for all these conditions.

AMS, HACE and HAPE

See the flow chart in Appendix 5 and the Lake Louise score in Appendix 6.

AMS (acute mountain sickness)

AMS varies from mild to severe and symptoms typically appear within 12 hours of the ascent.

Symptoms and signs

AMS presents with one or more of the following symptoms after a recent height gain:

- headache, typically throbbing and worse for bending or lying down (although in a few cases the headache may be mild or even absent)
- fatigue, tiredness, weakness, lassitude
- loss of appetite, or nausea, or vomiting
- dizziness, light-headedness.

HACE (high altitude cerebral edema)

AMS and HACE are two extremes of the same condition. Typically, symptoms and signs of AMS become worse and HACE develops. However, HACE may come on so quickly (in an hour or two) that the AMS stage is not noticed.

The important distinction between AMS and HACE is that with HACE there is also declining brain function with loss of physical coordination (**ataxia**) and an altered level of consciousness.

Symptoms and signs

A diagnosis of HACE is made when there has been a height gain in the last few days and, most importantly, there is impaired brain function.

- AMS-like symptoms may be present, such as headache, which can be severe and unresponsive to painkillers
- level of consciousness is declining and the victim cannot do simple mental tests
- as HACE progresses they become drowsy, semiconscious or unconscious
- loss of physical coordination (ataxia, clumsiness) occurs, they have difficulty with simple tasks such as tying shoelaces or packing their bag, and they may be staggering or falling over; they fail to perform any one of the tests for HACE (below)
- there may be nausea and/or vomiting, which may be severe and persistent

- personality changes may appear: disorientation, confusion, irritability, uncooperativeness, poor decision making
- they may wet themselves or be unable to pass urine
- hallucinations, blurred or double vision, seeing haloes around objects, fits or localized stroke signs may all occur but are less common.

TESTS FOR HACE

Failure to do, or *difficulty* in doing, or *refusal* to do any of these tests means the victim has HACE. If in doubt about their performance on the tests, compare with a healthy person. Repeat these tests to monitor progress.

- **Finger–nose test:** the victim repeatedly alternates between touching the tip of their nose with an index finger, then extending this arm to point into the distance (useful test if the victim is in a sleeping bag or cannot stand up). If they cannot do this quickly and accurately they have failed.

- **Heel-to-toe walking test:** the victim is asked to take several very small steps in a straight line (placing the heel of one foot in front of the toes of the other foot as they go) then a sharp about turn to retrace those steps. Reasonably flat ground is necessary and the victim should not be helped (but be prepared to catch them if they fall over). Excessive wobbling, flailing arms or falling over means failure.

- **Standing test:** the victim stands, feet together and arms by their sides, and then closes their eyes (the victim should not be helped, but be prepared to catch them if they fall over). Excessive wobbling or opening their eyes or falling over means failure.

- **Mental tests** are used to assess brain function. You must take into consideration pre-existing verbal/arithmetic skills and culture: it is a decline in ability over time that is significant. Examples of tests include 'spell your name backwards', 'take 3 from 50 and keep taking 3 from the result', or ask their birth date, about recent news events etc.

HAPE (high altitude pulmonary edema)

HAPE is the accumulation of fluid in the lungs. It is the most common cause of death due to altitude illness. HAPE may appear on its own without any preceding symptoms of AMS (this happens in about 50% of cases), or it may develop at the same time as AMS or HACE. Severe cases of HAPE may result, in the later stages, in the development of HACE.

HAPE may develop very rapidly (in 1 to 2 hours) or very gradually over days. It often develops during or after the second night at a new altitude. HAPE can even develop while descending from a higher altitude. HAPE is more likely to occur in people with chest infections or when the weather is very cold. It is easily mistaken for bronchitis/pneumonia/asthma. If you have the slightest doubt, treat for both.

Respiratory rate, clinical signs and general condition are the best indicators of progress, while pulse-oximetry may assist to gauge progress if extremities are warm.

Symptoms and signs

- A loss of physical performance with increased tiredness/fatigue, with or without a dry cough, is often the earliest sign of HAPE.
- Breathlessness (the most important sign of HAPE): in the early stages, the victim is more breathless with exercise and takes a little longer to get their breath back once resting. As HAPE progresses this gets worse until they are breathless at rest. They may be more breathless while lying flat and feel better sitting up.
- The respiratory rate at rest (measured after 5 minutes of sitting or lying down) increases as HAPE progresses, as does the pulse rate (at sea level, resting respiratory rate is 12–20 breaths/min at rest; at 6000m, normal acclimatized resting respiratory rate is approximately 25 breaths/min).
- As HAPE gets worse, the dry cough may start to bring up white frothy sputum. Later still, this frothy sputum may become blood-stained (pink or rust coloured).
- 'Wet' sounds (fine crackles) may be heard in the lungs when the victim breathes in deeply (place your ear on the bare skin of the victim's back below the shoulder blades, and even better, a hand's breadth below the armpit; compare with a healthy person). While wet sounds are conclusive, they may be difficult to hear or absent even in severe HAPE, so the absence of wet sounds does NOT exclude HAPE.
- There may be: a mild fever, a sense of inner cold, or pains in the chest or upper belly.
- Lips, tongue or nails may become blue.
- Eventually the victim becomes confused, drowsy, semiconscious, unconscious and will die if not treated urgently.

PART 3: Problems and their treatment

WHAT ELSE COULD IT BE?

If the illness comes on after four days at a new altitude and/or does not respond to descent, oxygen, dexamethasone and/or nifedipine, reconsider your diagnosis.

- HACE may be difficult to distinguish from: migraine, meningitis, diabetic coma, CO poisoning.
- HAPE may be difficult to distinguish from: pneumonia, pulmonary embolus (a blood clot from a DVT), heart attack, asthma, diabetic coma, hyperventilation (panic attack).

Unless absolutely sure, treat as HACE or HAPE (or both) PLUS your alternative diagnosis.

See also 'The high altitude quintet' above.

Treatment of altitude illness

If someone is ill at altitude after a recent height gain, carry out a full secondary survey (especially level of consciousness and respiratory rate), a 'Lake Louise Score' (Appendix 6) and the tests/examination for HACE and HAPE. Repeat all this regularly and note your findings.

Victims of altitude illness are often unable to look after themselves. It is imperative that the leader/doctor/companion makes decisions for them (eg ordering immediate descent), even if the victim disagrees.

- **Descent** is the most important and vital treatment of altitude illness. Prompt descent will begin to reverse the symptoms. Descend immediately if symptoms are severe, even if it means at night or in bad weather. The accepted therapeutic descent is 1000m or more but even as little as 500m can provide dramatic improvement. Resting at the same altitude is only acceptable if the victim has mild AMS with no single severe symptom, and is improving with treatment.

- **Oxygen:** give oxygen (bottled oxygen, portable oxygen separator or hyperbaric bag). Oxygen is lifesaving if the victim is too ill to move or when a meaningful descent is not immediately possible (due to flat or dangerous terrain, bad weather, not enough helpers to carry an unconscious victim, waiting for a helicopter etc). Oxygen will improve and/or stabilize the victim's condition before or during a descent. If you have a pulse-oximeter, aim for a PO2 of 90%.

HYPERBARIC BAGS AND BOTTLED OXYGEN

- **Hyperbaric bags** (PAC™, Certec™, Gamow™) are equivalent to a bottled oxygen flow rate of 2–4L/min. The victim will often breathe better (HAPE) or have less headache (HACE) with the head end of the bag propped up at least a 20° angle. If the victim is semi-conscious/unconscious, prop them in the safe airway position and keep a continuous watch on their position, condition and breathing and, if needed, deflate the bag and rectify any problems immediately. While treating a victim in a hyperbaric bag, short deflation breaks may be taken for examination or toilet purposes.

- **Bottled oxygen** allows higher flow rates.

Note: if both bottled oxygen and hyperbaric bag are available, a good option is to treat with high-flow oxygen (8+L/min) from the bottle while preparing to put the victim in the hyperbaric bag.

- Keep the victim warm, hydrated and fed.
- Avoid physical exertion as symptoms may worsen or reappear after treatment (rebound).
- Sit or prop them up in a semi-reclining position.
- Headache is best treated with ibuprofen (paracetamol is less risky above 5500m).
- Nausea or vomiting may need treating.
- Assisted breathing should be given if the victim is exhausted, hypothermic, has difficulty breathing, is turning blue or is deteriorating rapidly.

Drugs used for altitude illness

Refer to chart below for dosages.

- **Acetazolamide** (Diamox™) is used in prevention to speed up acclimatization. See 'Acetazolamide (Diamox™)', p. 39, for information and side effects.
- **Dexamethasone** is an effective treatment for HACE and for severe AMS. It may be given by mouth or (faster) by IM or IV. Only stop the dexamethasone after at least 3 days of treatment and once staying below

171

TREATMENT OF ALTITUDE ILLNESS

	Mild AMS (Lake Louise Score 3–5)	Moderate to severe AMS (Lake Louise Score 6 or more)	HACE	HAPE
DESCENT	Rest at the same (or lower) altitude until the symptoms clear (this will take a few hours to a few days)	Descend at least 500 to 1000m	*Descend immediately.* Descend as low as possible; at least 1000m or more	*Descend immediately.* Descend as low as possible; at least 1000m or more
OXYGEN • bottled	Consider 2L/min or more	2L/min or more	Start with higher flow and reduce as condition improves	Start with higher flow and reduce as condition improves
• hyperbaric bag	Until symptoms clear and then for an additional 30 minutes	Until symptoms clear and then for an additional 30 minutes	Typically for 4 hours or more	Typically for 6 to 8 hours or more
ACETAZOLAMIDE (diamox™)	Consider 125–250mg 12-hourly for the rest of the time at altitude if: a) Symptoms are still present at bedtime and an unavoidable ascent is due the following morning b) For 'slow acclimatizers', on tight schedules	250mg 12-hourly for the rest of the time at altitude		
DEXAMETHASONE May be given by mouth, IM or IV		For severe symptoms consider (8mg at once, then 4mg 6-hourly)	8mg at once then 4mg 6-hourly for the rest of the time at altitude	In severe cases 8mg at once then 4mg 6-hourly for the rest of the time at altitude
NIFEDIPINE Use only slow release S/R or modified release (MR) form				Consider 20–30mg 8 to 12-hourly, for at least 3 days. Give if victim is very ill, not improving or has to walk down.

2500m (this is because dexamethasone does mask the symptoms and signs of AMS/HACE, unlike acetazolamide). Tail off the dose slowly by giving the last 3 doses 12-hourly.

- **Nifedipine** is used in HAPE if there is no oxygen available, or the victim is seriously ill, or as an effective means of preventing recurrence of symptoms once oxygen is stopped. It is especially useful if the victim has to walk down. Nifedipine can drop the victim's blood pressure dramatically; to reduce this risk, use only the slow release (s/r or m/r) preparations of nifedipine, re-warm, rehydrate and avoid standing up suddenly.

Going back up again?

- Anyone seriously ill with HACE or HAPE needing oxygen, treatment in a hyperbaric bag, dexamethasone or nifedipine should descend immediately after treatment as, even if they feel completely recovered, as symptoms can rapidly reappear (rebound) with even mild exertion or further ascent. Oxygen and medication only buy time for descent.
- Cautious re-ascent may be considered once completely free of symptoms of HACE or HAPE for a week or two but the advice of a doctor qualified in mountain medicine should be sought first.
- If re-ascent is unavoidable (eg evacuation over high passes), give acetazolamide 250mg 12-hourly plus:
  - ▸ if the original problem was HACE, add dexamethasone (4mg 12-hourly)
  - ▸ if the problem was HAPE, add modified release nifedipine (20mg 12-hourly) plus dexamethasone (4mg 12-hourly).
- Give oxygen crossing passes or flying. Avoid long-haul jet flights until well.
- If symptoms of severe AMS disappear after descent and the victim is feeling well (and has been off dexamethasone for at least 3 days), they may try re-ascending slowly while continuing to take acetazolamide.

23. DROWNING AND DIVING PROBLEMS

Drowning (submersion)

If a person's head is under water (submersion) they eventually run out of breath and water is swallowed in large amounts which often results in vomiting and potential inhalation of stomach contents. With the brain and heart starved of oxygen, unconsciousness is followed by cardiac arrest and death.

- If the victim has fallen or dived in, been swept down rapids or dumped by a wave, assume they have a spinal injury.
- If they have been in cool or cold water, assume they are hypothermic.
- If they have been submerged in water for more than one hour, the chances of resuscitation are minimal (except for victims submerged in cold, clean water).

Management

This is one of the most dangerous situations for rescuers, so take great care not become a victim yourself (see 'In the water' p. 26).

- Get the victim out of the water, trying to keep them as horizontal as possible (the vertical position may kill them).
- If there is no sign of life, start CPR: do not waste time trying to empty water from their lungs.
- Give oxygen once breathing is re-established.
- **'Car park collapse'**: If someone has suffered a drowning event (especially if they lost consciousness at any point), their condition will be unstable for some hours afterwards. Check their vital signs regularly and evacuate by stretcher to medical help. If evacuation is not possible, keep them still and under observation for 24 hours. Allowing them to exercise too soon may result in death.

Diving

On surfacing, divers are usually dehydrated and mildly hypothermic.

There are specific problems associated with scuba diving, and knowing the basics of how to prevent, recognise and deal with them is vital. Any symptoms or signs, however mild or strange, especially within an hour of resurfacing, should be taken to be dive-related.

What follows is a much simplified outline of the commonest problems. Seek expert advice as soon as possible (see Appendix 10 – 'Water').

Barotrauma

This is experienced during descent when hollow organs (middle ear, sinuses, lungs) suffer the results of pressure changes.

Symptoms and signs

These include pain, deafness, ringing, vertigo in one or both ears due to damage to eardrum, middle or inner ear. Blood may appear in the ear drum. Facial pain or nosebleed from sinus trauma may occur.

Treatment

No diving for 4 weeks after a ruptured eardrum, and preferably not until after a medical check. Treat ear, throat or sinus infections and congestion.

Nitrogen narcosis

This occurs at a depth of 30m or more and can cause death by clouding good judgement.

Symptoms and signs

Euphoria, light-headedness, slow reflexes, poor judgement, hallucinations, unconsciousness.

Treatment

Early recognition, buddying up and appropriate ascent.

Decompression illness (DCI)

DCI symptoms usually appear within one hour of surfacing but may be delayed by up to 48 hours. It is caused by formation of nitrogen gas bubbles in tissues (decompression sickness) and arteries (cerebral arterial gas embolism causing the neurological problems). It is not necessary to make a definitive diagnosis, but early recognition of symptoms and prompt action is.

Symptoms and signs

Symptoms and signs may be obvious or hardly noticeable.

- Headache, loss of appetite, tiredness
- Painful muscles and joints ('**the bends**'), which typically involves shoulders and elbows, but may affect any joint or muscle; abdominal pain may also occur
- Lungs and breathing: shortness of breath, chest pain and cough, with or without blood

175

- Nervous system: clumsiness, staggering, falling, change in level of consciousness, coma, paralysis, weakness, difficulty swallowing, tingling, numbness, memory loss
- Bladder and bowels may not work properly

Treatment
If any of the above symptoms appear between surfacing and 48 hours afterwards, arrange for immediate evacuation to a dive medicine centre/decompression chamber. Seek medical advice. Act even if the symptoms and signs are mild, as they may progress.

- BLS, keep victim horizontal.
- Give high flow 100% oxygen.
- Re-warm and rehydrate (normal saline solution).
- If evacuating by plane, helicopter or road, try to keep below 150m higher than the altitude where the dive took place to avoid worsening the problem.

24. INFECTIOUS DISEASES

There are many serious infectious diseases: research those prevalent in the area to be visited.

It may be impossible to find out exactly what the problem is: a good secondary survey, repeated regularly, is the only way to get some idea of the cause and severity and when to evacuate. Below is a simple guide to help.

See Chapter 1, 'Preventing spread of infection', 'Preventing mosquito-borne diseases' and 'Preventing other insect-borne diseases'.

Mosquito-borne diseases

Malaria
This deadly disease occurs in most of Africa, Southeast Asia, South and Central America and in the Himalayas below 1000m. The incubation period for malaria is usually a week or two, but may be many months depending on the malaria strain. Preventative medication is not 100% effective and may delay the onset of symptoms. Some strains of malaria are deadly and can kill in 24 hours. Early diagnosis is important so find a doctor who can make the correct diagnosis by blood testing (malaria self-test kits are now available).

Symptoms and signs
- Fever, with chills and sweats; the illness is often mild to begin with, but eventually the victim becomes very ill
- Headache and muscle aches that may come and go with no obvious cause
- Possible nausea, vomiting, abdominal pain or jaundice
- Eventual reduction in level of consciousness, with confusion, drowsiness and finally coma

Treatment
Only self-treat if there has been exposure to malaria for more than a week, you are more than 24 hours from medical help, AND there is a fever over 38°C. Do not use the same antibiotic for treatment as the one taken for prevention.

Dengue fever
This occurs in most of the tropical/subtropical regions of the world and is particularly common in North India. Its incubation period is around 10

days and the illness lasts a week or so. There is no specific treatment so avoid bites. It can be difficult to differentiate from malaria.

Symptoms and signs
- Sudden onset of fever with severe headache
- Severe pain in muscles/bones (hence its common name **'break bone fever'**)
- Possible vomiting and possible slight rash
- In the severe haemorrhagic form of the disease, possible death from internal bleeding. This is more likely with subsequent infections

Treatment
Give painkillers (paracetamol or codeine). As there is a potential for internal bleeding, do NOT give aspirin, ibuprofen and other NSAIDs.

Yellow fever
Yellow fever is a serious haemorrhagic viral illness found in South America and tropical Africa. Vaccination is essential. Avoid being bitten.

Symptoms and signs are similar to dengue fever, but the skin and eye white may turn yellow. Evacuate.

Japanese encephalitis
This deadly viral infection of the brain is found in an arc from India through Southeast Asia, Indonesia, China, Korea, Japan, the western Pacific and eastern Russia. Vaccination is available. Avoid being bitten. Symptoms are as for meningitis but antibiotics do not work on the virus. If in doubt treat as meningitis.

Zika virus
This virus is presently found in many tropical countries but appears to be spreading. It can be sexually transmitted. It causes mild flu-like symptoms lasting up to a week. Unfortunately it can cause foetal abnormalities in pregnant women. There is no vaccination or definitive treatment. Avoid being bitten.

Tick-borne diseases

Apart from being a nuisance, tick bites may transmit a wide range of nasty diseases, such as Lyme disease, Rocky Mountain spotted fever, relapsing fever, Q fever, tick typhus, tick paralysis and tick encephalitis. See 'Preventing other insect-borne diseases' p. 19.

Early recognition and treatment with antibiotics (if appropriate) is essential. If ticks are suspected or likely, carry out a thorough daily whole body search for ticks – including belly button, ear canals and all hairy places - and remove. See 'Ticks', p. 127.

- **Tick-borne rickettsial diseases:** rash, tiredness, fever, weakness, severe headaches, muscle pains, swollen lymph glands. Give antibiotics (Appendix 2)
- **Lyme disease**: flu-like symptoms, rash (sometimes a typical bulls eye rash may appear around the bite), joint and muscle pain and weakness, headache. It can become chronic. Give antibiotics (Appendix 2)
- **Tick encephalitis**: found in Central and Eastern Europe and Russia, it is viral and vaccination is available. Symptoms and signs resemble those of meningitis and treatment is limited to general nursing care. However, if meningitis cannot be excluded, give antibiotics as for meningitis (Appendix 2)
- **Australian paralysis tick disease**: restlessness, irritability and pins and needles in hands and feet may be followed by paralysis. Give supportive treatment as recovery gradually occurs

In all the above diseases, chronic symptoms will need to be dealt with by a doctor.

Diseases from contaminated water

These are best prevented by vaccination and strict hygiene (see 'Preventing diarrhoea and food poisoning', p. 14).

Typhoid
This serious bacterial illness is often difficult to recognize.

Symptoms and signs
- Feels and looks ill with increasing fever with shivering chills and a relatively slow pulse
- Headache, sore throat
- A possible faint rash on the body.
- Possible diarrhoea with 'pea-soup' stools.
- Possibly semiconscious, disoriented and confused

The condition lasts for 2 to 3 weeks and the victim may die.

Treatment
- Give antibiotics (Appendix 2).

Hepatitis A

This viral infection of the liver has an incubation time of 10 days to 6 weeks. It may be so mild as to be unnoticeable, especially in children, or severe enough to cause death, especially in older people. Hepatitis A occurs worldwide but is most common in developing tropical/subtropical countries. The victim is highly infectious up to 10 days after the onset of jaundice. Vaccination is recommended.

Symptoms and signs
- Victim feels unwell, fever and flu-like symptoms
- Nausea and vomiting (sometimes severe), loss of appetite
- Possible **jaundice** (yellow eyes and skin, itchy skin, dark yellow urine and white stools)

Treatment
- Bed rest with a low fat, high carbohydrate (sugars and starches) and fruit diet
- Alcohol and other recreational drugs should be avoided until blood tests show normal liver function or, in the absence of medical advice, for 6 months after recovery

Other infectious diseases

Meningitis

Certain viruses or bacteria may infect the covering (meninges) of the brain. Vaccination can prevent some epidemic forms (eg meningococcal meningitis).

Symptoms and signs
- Fever with severe headache and intolerance of bright lights
- Neck stiffness: pain on attempting to bring knees up to chest or place chin on chest
- Possibly a typical purple rash that does NOT lose its colour with pressure (use a clear glass to apply pressure and look through it to see whether the rash disappears)
- Possible fits and vomiting
- Confusion leading to unconsciousness and death in severe cases

Treatment
Give antibiotics (Appendix 2).

Rabies
This deadly viral brain fever is found in many countries worldwide and is transmitted by a bite of an infected animal (eg dog, monkey, bat or human). The incubation period is usually three to 20 weeks but can be years.

Symptoms and signs
- From an early stage: tiredness, fever, headache, sore throat, nausea, abdominal pain
- Mental changes: anxiety, agitation and irritability, depression
- After a week or so: either progressive paralysis with difficulty talking, swallowing, breathing or a very agitated, aggressive state with possible fits

Treatment
- Clean the bites thoroughly.
- The victim must seek urgent post-exposure vaccination and treatment (even if they had pre-exposure vaccination).

25. EYES, EARS AND MOUTH

Eyes

Common eye problems are usually easy to diagnose and treat. Rarer but more dangerous problems are generally harder to diagnose and will require urgent evacuation.

Conjunctivitis

This infection of the 'white' of the eye (conjunctiva) often starts in one eye but usually spreads to the other. It is very contagious.

The white of the eye is inflamed, red, feels gritty and possibly feels sore or itchy. Pus may develop with the eyelids sticking together and pus accumulating in the corner of the eye, especially noticeable on waking up.

Treatment

Make sure that there is no foreign object in the eye. If this is not a possibility and no foreign object is seen:

- remove contact lenses
- if no pus is present, this is probably **viral conjunctivitis** that will clear up in 10 days without antibiotics
- if pus is present, gently wash it away with drinkable water before inserting antibiotic eye ointment/drops (a squeeze/2 drops, 3-hourly for one day, reducing to 6-hourly for at least two more days).

Infected eyelid

This may be a 'stye' (small, localized abscess) or **blepharitis** (a more generalized infection). The eyelid is inflamed and pus may appear at the lid margin.

Treatment

- Hot compresses (eg a wrung out used tea bag once it has cooled a little) to the eyelid several times daily
- Antibiotic eye drops/ointment as for conjunctivitis

Infection of the eyeball or around the eye

Infections of the ball of the eye itself (**orbital cellulitis**), especially if it has been injured, or of tissue around the eye (peri-orbital cellulitis) are serious conditions.

- The eye or tissues around the eye are infected and swollen, red and painful, with limitation of eye movement. The sinus areas may be tender and the victim unwell.

- Vision may be affected and meningitis and blindness may occur if the infection spreads to the brain.

Treatment
Give antibiotics (Appendix 2). Give nasal decongestant/spray. Evacuate if not settling rapidly and completely.

Sudden loss of vision
This has various causes and urgent evacuation is indicated. The only possible exception to evacuation is a **retinal haemorrhage** in a high altitude climber (where a sudden localized partial loss of vision occurs), as resting at a lower altitude will slowly fix the problem.

Solitary red eye
If one eye only becomes red, inflamed and/or painful without the possibility of a foreign object or trauma, it may be a dangerous eye condition such as **iritis**, **corneal ulcer** or **glaucoma**. Increasing pain, severe pain, intolerance to bright light, blurry vision or loss of vision are indications to seek urgent medical advice. Less serious causes of red eye (such as subconjunctival bleed) are usually painless, mild, self-limiting and will gradually improve.

Superficial foreign object or chemicals in the eye

Chemicals
As soon as possible use the cleanest water available to flush out the chemical for 20 minutes. If the other eye is unaffected, keep the draining water out of it.

Foreign body

Symptoms and signs
- The affected eye is red and watering.
- It feels like there is something gritty in the eye, or it is very painful.
- Blinking and moving the eye makes the pain worse.
- Pain may cause intense spasm of the eyelids which cannot be opened, making inspection difficult.

Treatment
- Take your time, and put the victim in a comfortable, semi-reclining position. Wash your hands. Using your best light, stand behind the victim

to look under the lower lid by pulling it out and asking the victim to look up first and then from one side to the other. Now stand in front of the victim, take hold of the upper eyelid by the lashes and gently pull it back over a cotton bud, asking them to look down. If you cannot see anything, try again using a magnifying glass/reading glasses.

- If eyelid spasm makes it impossible to open the eye, insert 1 or 2 drops of eye anaesthetic and then proceed (**Note:** once anaesthetized, you must keep the eye closed or well covered with a clean pad to prevent injury from any remaining, or new, foreign object until feeling returns after a few hours. If vision is needed for self-rescue, use sunglasses or, better still, goggles).
- Whether you can see the foreign object or not, try washing it out of the eye with clean, boiled and cooled water, or normal saline solution (chlorinated tap water can be used but will turn the eye red):
  ▸ open and close the eye repeatedly while immersed in a small container of the liquid, or
  ▸ let it gently trickle across the surface of the eye.
- If washing doesn't work, try gently brushing the foreign object off using a corner of gauze, clean handkerchief or cotton bud (never use tweezers, needles, pins or anything sharp).
- If the foreign object is removed, insert antibiotic eye ointment (12-hourly for 24 hours).
- If the victim still feels there is something in their eye, repeat your examination and treatments, insert antibiotic eye ointment as above.
- If pain and the sensation of 'something in the eye' do not now settle in a few hours, gets worse, if vision becomes blurry or if there is a foreign object you cannot remove, insert antibiotic eye ointment 12-hourly and pad the eye (or both eyes if pain due to eye movement is a problem). Give painkillers and evacuate.

Penetrating object in the eye

A splinter or flying fragments from chipped stone or metal can get stuck in the tough membrane of the eye, or go right through this membrane into the eyeball (this is easily missed, with serious consequences).

Symptoms and signs
- Pain (or no pain), vision may be affected, watering eye
- Obvious bleeding or injury and/or an obvious protruding object

There may be no signs and symptoms, especially with deeply penetrating high velocity, tiny metallic objects.

Treatment

If there is a protruding object:

- do not touch the eye or the object; do not put anything in the eye
- apply a ring pad dressing (Fig 14.2) around the eye, resting on the bones. Pad both eyes closed (if possible) and encourage the victim to keep their eyes still to reduce damage (you have to cover the good eye to do this)
- prevent/treat vomiting and coughing
- give painkillers and evacuate.

If there is no protruding object but the MOI suggests that deep penetration has occurred, evacuate as this often painless injury may eventually cause blindness in both eyes.

Dry eyes and contact lenses problems

Dry eyes occur in very dry and windy environments: lubricant drops and sunglasses usually ease the problem.

Contact lenses may cause pain if left in too long: lubricant drops, sunglasses and removal usually fixes the problem.

Snow blindness (photokeratitis)

Ultraviolet light (UV) reflected from snow, ice, quartz rock or even water can 'burn' the cornea/conjunctiva of the eye. This is a crippling injury and can immobilize the victim for 24 hours.

Symptoms and signs

The eyes become red, watery and very painful, and cannot tolerate light. The victim is often agitated/afraid.

Treatment

- Stop the victim from rubbing their eyes; apply cold compresses and gentle pressure. Reassure them they will recover.
- Give painkillers (ibuprofen for inflammation, adding paracetamol or codeine if needed).
- In severe cases, insert antibiotic eye ointment and anaesthetic eye drops, pad eyes closed (both preferably) for 12 hours.
- Do NOT insert steroid drops.
- Snow blind mountaineers may have to use anaesthetic eye drops (one drop 2 to 4-hourly) to allow them to climb out of danger (use goggles to prevent foreign objects, eg dust, getting into the eyes, as these will not be felt until the anaesthetic wears off some hours later).

185

Ears

Infections of the outer and middle ear may be hard to tell apart: if in doubt treat as both.

Infection of the outer ear
This may be a generalized infection of the canal or a localized **boil/abscess**. It is often caused by wet ears after swimming. Using alcohol, vinegar drops or Aquaear™ will prevent most infections.

Symptoms and signs
- From an early stage, itching (at this point the victim must not scratch)
- Red, painful ear and possibly smelly pus discharging from the ear
- Pain when pulling on the earlobe (pulling does not cause pain in a middle ear infection)
- A boil may occur in the ear canal; this is very painful, especially when the earlobe is pulled

Treatment

Simple infection
- Very gently wash out as much discharge as possible using a dilute solution of betadine, then dry with a wisp of cotton wool or toilet paper.
- Lay the victim on their side and fill the infected ear with antibiotic ointment/eardrops (or a combined antibiotic/anti-inflammatory preparation such as Sofradex HC™) for 20 minutes. **Note:** chloramphenicol eye ointment may be used if you have nothing else.
- Continue the eardrops/ointment (4 drops into the ear 6-hourly for up to 7 days), gently cleaning the ear canal before each application of the eardrops/ointment.
- Once healed, keep the ear dry.

Severe infection
If the eardrops/ointment are not working (or not available), or the victim is ill or pain is severe or redness and tenderness are spreading around and behind the ear, add antibiotics (Appendix 2).

Infection in the middle ear
This often follows a cold or a sore throat.

Symptoms and signs
- A feeling of blockage, dullness or deafness in the ear, and possible fever and pain which may be severe (but pulling the ear is not painful)
- Eventually the eardrum may burst, which results in relief from pain and discharge of pus from the ear. Hearing is reduced but returns when the eardrum heals after four weeks. Keep the ear dry until then

Treatment
- Use a nasal decongestant and steam inhalations.
- Give painkillers (ibuprofen and/or paracetamol).
- If the victim is in increasing pain, give antibiotics (Appendix 2).

Foreign object in the ear or nose

Something in the ear
A strong light may tempt out a **live insect**; if not try gently washing it out using a syringe (no needle) filled with vegetable oil or lukewarm drinkable water.
Button batteries need urgent removal by a specialist.
Do NOT syringe ears if there is a perforated eardrum. Do not use water to flush out a seed as it may expand.

Object in the nose
Blow in the victim's mouth while closing the unobstructed nostril.

Mouth and teeth (contributed by Dr Renée Farrar)

When examining teeth, use a good head torch, gloves and spectacles.

Lost fillings
If a filling falls out, or becomes loose, remove it to stop food debris collecting under it, as it may cause infection. Treat as for toothache.

Toothache
This is usually due to a hole in the enamel of the tooth, caused by decay, with resulting inflammation/infection. Pain comes and goes and is made worse by hot/cold food or drinks.

If there is no infection:

Treatment
- Dry the hole thoroughly and place a rolled up gauze in the space between the cheek and the gum to catch saliva.
- Press a tiny blob of Cavit™ mixed with clove oil into the bottom of the hole.
- Fill the hole, using either:
  ‣ a temporary filling of Cavit™: tell the victim to bite down gently while it is still setting, to avoid biting discomfort due to an overfilled hole;
  ‣ OR cotton wool soaked with clove oil (replacing it when necessary);
  ‣ OR sugar free chewing gum.
- Give ibuprofen plus paracetamol for pain, and a soft diet for three days, with salt-water mouth rinses or chlorhexidine mouthwash three times a day.

If there is infection (**tooth abscess**):
There will be pain, typically throbbing and intense, tenderness, a bad taste (and often smell) in the mouth and possible swelling of the gum (a **gumboil**).

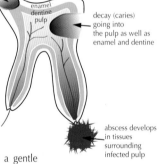

decay going into enamel and dentine

enamel
dentine
pulp

decay (caries) going into the pulp as well as enamel and dentine

abscess develops in tissues surrounding infected pulp

Fig 25.1 Tooth abscess

Treatment
- Start antibiotics (Appendix 2).
- Make a small nick in the gumboil to drain the pus.
- Remove any filling if you can then clean the hole with a gentle toothpick and wash with saline or chlorhexidine mouthwash.
- Leave the hole to drain. Tell patient not to bite on this side. Any facial swelling needs to be treated with antibiotics. Don't fill up a draining tooth abscess – it may cause a buildup of infection.
- If ill or not settled evacuate urgently.

Severe infections of the mouth
These can affect the gums, tongue or cheeks. This is painful, and the breath smells bad. See 'Respiratory tract infections', p. 160.

Treatment
- Use regular mouthwashes (chlorhexidine or salt water), plus a soft diet to minimize chewing.
- If there is no improvement or pain is severe, give antibiotics (Appendix 2).
- If swallowing or breathing become difficult, evacuate.

Damaged/broken teeth
A blow to the face has to be hard to damage or knock out a tooth, so always check for facial fractures and head injury as well.

Treatment
- Paint the exposed surface of the broken tooth with clove oil, or suck on a clove, or apply a thin layer of Duraphat™ (a concentrated fluoride paste to be used sparingly – avoid swallowing and apply as a thin layer, with no eating for 30 minutes). This should reduce acute sensitivity from cold and hot things.
- If a tooth is knocked out, or is loose, do not scrub clean (if it needs cleaning, ask the victim to suck it clean, or use milk or normal saline solution). If you can get to a dentist, store the tooth in a plastic bag with some of the patient's saliva. In a remote situation, try to put it back into the socket as quickly as possible. Then add a tin foil splint fashioned around the teeth like a mouth guard. Seek dental help once available. Do not attempt this procedure if the victim has a lowered level of consciousness as they may inhale the tooth or splint.
- If the socket won't stop bleeding, bite on a rolled gauze for 20 minutes. If this doesn't work, stitch the socket closed, removing the stitches three days later.

Serious dental infection
Dental, facial or throat infections can easily spread and cause life-threatening infection that compromises breathing/eyesight.

Warning signs
- Swelling that leads to an eye closing
- Difficulty opening the mouth or any neck swelling
- Fever, shivering, loss of appetite, nausea and vomiting

Treatment
Give antibiotics (Appendix 2) as for tooth abscess. See 'Facial injuries' (p. 109) and 'Infection of the eyeball or around the eye' (p. 182).

26. SKIN PROBLEMS

Rashes

A rash may be caused by infection, allergy or inflammation. It may be difficult to work out the cause even after a complete secondary survey with a thorough medical history.

General treatment
- Do not scratch as breaking the skin's barrier may cause a bacterial secondary skin infection; cover with a light dressing if necessary.
- Keep wet rashes dry, and dry rashes moist.
- If you cannot work out the cause, stop all recently started medication (if safe to do so), apply cold compresses and/or calamine lotion and wait.

Allergies
See 'Side effects and allergic reactions', p. 37 and 'Allergy' p. 206. There are many causes of allergic skin rashes, common examples are contact with chemicals, latex and some plants.

Eczema (dermatitis)
Patches of inflamed skin become red, itchy, scaly, dry or wet and can take many forms. It is usually a recurrent problem for the victim, who should be able to identify it. Treat as for allergy and, if dry, add a moisturizer.

Impetigo ('school sores')
This is a highly contagious superficial skin infection that often starts as small pus-filled blisters that rapidly break down into areas of weeping red skin.

Treatment
- Clean with disinfectant solution, dry and apply antibiotic ointment (8-hourly for up to 7 days).
- If antibiotic ointment alone is not working or the infection is extensive, give antibiotics (Appendix 2).

Fleas, bed bugs
See 'Bed bugs, fleas', p. 127.

Fungal infection

These appear as a slowly spreading patch(es) on the skin with an itchy, red edge and a paler centre (**ringworm**). Moist hot areas (groin, armpits, under breasts and genitals) are especially vulnerable and a painful shiny red rash may develop. When between toes, the skin is cracked/painful.

Trench foot is a painful fungal condition due to prolonged wet feet and socks.

Treatment

Keep clean and dry, applying antifungal cream (continuing for a week after the rash disappears).

Scabies

This is a very itchy rash caused by a small burrowing mite. It is usually caught after close contact with infected people or their furniture.

Symptoms and signs

- The rash spreads slowly over days or weeks on the arms, legs and body, especially the groin and between the fingers. It never affects the face. The victim constantly scratches, worse at night.
- Tracks under the skin can sometimes be seen with the naked eye or a magnifying glass.

Treatment

- Apply benzyl benzoate or permethrin cream (Lyclear™).
- The itch often increases after treatment; treat this itch as an allergy.

Shingles

A painful area occurs on one side of the body or face followed a short time later by a red rash with blisters. The victim feels unwell, the pain may be severe and persistent. The rash will settle after a week or two. If the rash affects an eye, this is serious and needs evacuation for specialist care.

Treatment

Give adequate pain relief, clean and dress the rash. If available, start an antiviral antibiotic (acyclovir) within 72 hours of the onset of symptoms.

PART 3: Problems and their treatment

Viral illnesses

Many viral illnesses such as chicken pox, rubella or measles (a nasty illness that can have serious consequences) can cause rashes. They often start with a fever, runny nose and sore throat, the typical rashes appearing later.

Treatment

Rest, hydrate, treat any symptoms, apply calamine lotion.

Prickly Heat
See p. 142.

Other skin problems

Boils and abscesses

Bacterial infection causes boils in the skin or abscesses under the skin, starting off as a small hard lump that turns red and painful, then gradually softens and enlarges as the infected tissue dies. With time it will turn yellow as pus surfaces, ready to discharge.

Treatment

- Apply hot compresses (use a cloth soaked in hot water and wrung out) to bring the infection to the surface, where it will break and discharge. Apply for 15 minutes every hour. Magnesium sulphate paste applied regularly has the same effect.
- If the boil looks yellowish at its softest point and looks unlikely to burst without help, it can be opened with a sterilized scalpel or very sharp knife (you may need to anaesthetize the skin) or warm up a glass jar in hot water and place it upside down over the boil: as the warm air inside the bottle cools down creating suction, the pus is sucked out.
- Once open, wear protective gloves to squeeze the pus out, using a finger to enlarge the hole if necessary (this is painful but important).
- Prevent the hole from healing over by gently packing wet sterile gauze into the hole and taping it in place. Replace this packing every 24 hours until the cavity heals, usually in 3 or 4 days.
- If the victim is in pain or the skin infection spreads, treat with antibiotics as for wound infection (Appendix 2). **Note:** antibiotics will not fully treat a boil or abscess unless it is draining. If the victim is feverish and unwell, see 'Septicaemia', p. 117.

Polar hands

'Polar hands' is the term used to describe painful cracks in the skin of the fingertips and around the nails. It can also affect the heels. It is caused by cold and dry conditions.

Treatment

- Use moisturizers, especially those high in lanolin, and rub down thickened layers of dead skin regularly.
- Clean cracks thoroughly with disinfectant solution and dry.
- Fill the cracks with superglue or squeeze in a little antibiotic ointment, hold the skin edges firmly together with adhesive tape and keep dry.

27. GENDER-SPECIFIC PROBLEMS AND STIs

Women

Cystitis (bladder infection)
This is quite common in women (rare in men). The cause, especially in women, is usually unknown; however, lack of hygiene, dehydration, sexual activity or STIs may be responsible.

Symptoms and signs
- Frequent, burning and/or painful urination; urine may be discoloured, smelly or bloodstained and often passed in small amounts
- Dull pain in lower abdomen or a sense of fullness (without fever)

Treatment
- Drink lots of water (at least 3 litres in 24 hours).
- Give antibiotics (Appendix 2). Women who suffer recurrent cystitis often carry a course of antibiotics to treat themselves.
- Improve hygiene in the genital area; wash with soap and water.

Vaginal fungal infection (thrush, candida)
This unpleasant infection may be caused by oral antibiotic treatments, hot climates, poor hygiene or sexual activity.

Symptoms and signs
- Painful, itchy or burning vagina or entrance to the vagina
- Possible thick white vaginal discharge, typically with little or no smell
- The infection may spread to the surrounding skin if neglected

Treatment
- Apply an antifungal cream externally 12-hourly for 7 days.
- Insert antifungal cream into the vagina at night for 3 nights: 'inject' a 5ml syringe (no needle!) full of antifungal cream, or apply antifungal cream liberally to a tampon and insert for 8 hours.
- If the discharge does not improve with treatment, suspect a STI.

Kidney infection
This serious infection may be due to untreated cystitis, or there may be no obvious cause. See also 'Serious abdominal problems' p. 155.

Symptoms and signs
- Fever and chills
- Back pain below the rib margins (may be both sides or one-sided)
- Possible nausea, vomiting, abdominal pain and symptoms and signs of cystitis (above)

Treatment
- Rest and drink water (500ml every 30 minutes for 2 hours, followed by 4 litres every 24 hours).
- Give antibiotics (Appendix 2).

Pelvic infection
May be caused by an intra-uterine contraceptive device (coil), STIs, or there may be no obvious cause. It can be very difficult to diagnose or differentiate from other abdominal problems. See 'Kidney infection' above and 'Serious abdominal problems', p. 155.

Symptoms and signs
- Feeling and looking unwell, fever
- Lower abdominal pain, low back pain, lower abdominal tenderness, with possible nausea and vomiting
- Possible menstrual problems (heavy, painful, early, smelly) or a vaginal discharge that is smelly

Treatment
Give antibiotics (Appendix 2).

Period pains, mid-cycle pain
Pain related to a woman's period may occur just before and/or during menstruation, or halfway between periods (mid-cycle pain). The victim has usually had this before.

Symptoms and signs
Sharp, lower abdominal pain that can sometimes be felt in the low back and upper thighs. This pain can be quite severe and resemble appendicitis, pelvic infection (above) or tubal pregnancy, but there is no fever and it eventually settles. Repeat the secondary survey until you have a diagnosis.

PART 3: Problems and their treatment

Treatment
- Rest, avoid coffee and try hot water bottles to the stomach or back.
- Give painkillers (ibuprofen 800mg once and then 400mg 8-hourly; add paracetamol if severe).

Heavy menstrual bleeding
A woman can have very heavy periods, with or without clots, which can last longer than normal. Pain may be present. See 'Tubal (ectopic) pregnancy', below.

Treatment
Rest; avoid coffee. Ibuprofen (400mg 6-hourly) may help. Seek medical advice if not settling.

Childbirth in a wilderness setting
The vast majority of births proceed normally and most women know what to expect. Anxiety may be the biggest problem in a remote setting, so a calm and competent manner is important. A normal labour will last approximately 12–20 hours from start to finish. First there is usually a small show of blood and mucus, and later a rush of 'water' and increasingly frequent contractions. Just before the birth the desire to push becomes very marked and pain may be severe with shouting/screaming (this is quite normal).

You will need: a clean blanket, cloth or towel to wrap the baby; hot water to wash your hands; a face mask; a plastic sheet or tarp to cover sleeping mats and make a birthing surface; a warm room or tent; and privacy. Keep anyone with a sore throat or skin infection away (even the baby's father or close relatives).

- Before handling the baby during the delivery or touching the mother's genital area, scrub your hands with hot water, soap and a nailbrush for 5 minutes. Preferably wear sterile surgical gloves (these are not essential but your bare hands must be scrupulously clean), and roll up your sleeves.
- Allow the mother to assume her most comfortable position; initially walking around, then maybe kneeling on all fours, squatting, lying on their side (best positions take advantage of gravity).
- Give teaspoons of honey for energy, and sips of water between contractions (remind the mother to urinate every two hours). Massage her lower back for pain relief; reassure and encourage her to focus on her breathing.

- Do not interfere with the birth process (ie do not hold the baby back, nor pull on it to speed things up). As soon as the face is delivered, wipe any mucus from the baby's nose and mouth.
- Once completely out, the baby usually cries straight away. If it does not, lie it on its side and massage the body firmly toward the head; flicking the soles of the feet may also stimulate a cry.
- Wrap the baby up warmly including the head and give it to the mother to cuddle. Keep them both warm.
- Massage the mother's lower abdomen gently to encourage the uterus to contract and place the baby on the breast. Both these actions reduce the vaginal bleeding that occurs after the birth.
- The mother may be mildly shocked.
- Clean the mother's genital area with clean water and apply sanitary pads or a boiled, dried towel.
- The placenta will deliver naturally within 10 to 90 minutes; do not pull on the cord.
- Cut the umbilical cord when you are ready (at least 5 minutes after delivery). Tie sterilized/disinfected string tightly around the umbilical cord: two ties at 10 and 15cm from the baby then a second tie at 20cm. Cut between these last ties (15 and 20cm) with sterilized scissors. Cover the cut end with a sterile dressing.
- The placenta should be checked carefully to see whether it is complete: if it is not, evacuate urgently for surgery.

Miscarriage

Miscarriage occurs frequently, usually in the early stages of pregnancy. Heavy bleeding and pain are sometimes accompanied by the passage of recognizable foetal parts/membranes. Complications can be life-threatening heavy bleeding and infection. Treat for shock and as for pelvic infection.

Tubal (ectopic) pregnancy

This is where the embryo develops in the narrow tube leading from the ovary to the uterus in early pregnancy. The tube will eventually burst causing severe abdominal pain due to bleeding and peritonitis. This is deadly without surgical treatment.

Symptoms and signs

- Missed period, irregular vaginal bleeding
- Early signs of pregnancy: breast tenderness, nausea, frequency of urination

- Pain and symptoms similar to those of appendicitis but on either side
- Worsening symptoms and shock

Treatment
Treat shock, evacuate urgently. If evacuation is delayed, treat as appendicitis (just in case it is).

Toxic shock syndrome
A rare condition, toxic shock occurs in menstruating women using tampons. Poor hygiene and super absorbent tampons left in place for more than 12 hours promote the growth of bacteria.

Symptoms and signs
Sudden onset of high fever, shock, vomiting, diarrhoea, muscle aches, rash.

Treatment
Remove tampon, treat as shock and septicaemia.

Men

Occasionally men suffer from moderate to severe pain in their testicles. The two commonest causes are twisted testicle and infection of the tubes behind the testicle and/or the testicle itself.

Twisted testicle
The victim (usually a teenager/young man) experiences a sudden onset of severe pain spreading from a red swollen testicle to their groin, and sometimes the lower abdomen, often with nausea and vomiting.

Treatment
- Evacuate for urgent surgical treatment to prevent death of the part (within 4 hours).
- If evacuation is delayed treat as for appendicitis, keeping the part cool.

Infection of the testicles and/or its veins
This can be can be very hard to tell from a twisted testicle. It comes on slowly; the victim feels unwell with a fever. The testicle is swollen red and tender, and the pain is eased by supporting the scrotum (unlike twisted testicle).

Treatment
- Give antibiotics as for prostatitis (Appendix 2) and support (2 pairs of underpants).

Prostatitis

This is an infection of the prostate gland. There is pain in the perineum (between anus and scrotum) and the victim feels unwell. Sitting (especially on a saddle) is painful.

Treatment
- Give painkillers (ibuprofen 400mg 8-hourly) and antibiotics (Appendix 2).

Sexually transmitted infections (STIs)

If anyone develops any of the symptoms below, a medical opinion should be sought as soon as possible, and sex should be avoided until diagnosed and treated. If medical advice is not available, the following notes may help.
- STIs may be a cause of cystitis or pelvic infection.
- **Vaginal discharge** may be caused by **Trichomonas vaginalis** (thick yellow discharge, itchiness and urinary discomfort). Give antibiotics (Appendix 2); see 'Vaginal fungal infection', p. 194.
- **Chlamydia** in men is often without symptoms, but women may experience cystitis-like symptoms or pelvic symptoms similar to a mild pelvic infection. Treat victim and partner with antibiotics (Appendix 2).
- **Gonorrhoea** may cause a drip of pus from penis or urethra, or symptoms like cystitis. Give antibiotics (Appendix 2).
- **Hepatitis B** is transmitted sexually or via blood-to-blood contact. Symptoms and treatment are similar to those of hepatitis A.
- **Warts** on sex organs and around the anus appear as crops of flat or filament-like soft growths. This is non-urgent but requires treatment when home.
- **Genital herpes** appears as painful sores, blisters on sexual parts. Apply acyclovir cream, give painkillers.
- **HIV/Aids** or **syphilis** may cause unexplained skin rashes, flu-like symptoms or ulcers of the skin or the genitals.

28. OTHER PROBLEMS

Headache and migraine

Headache
There are many possible causes of headache, such as heat exhaustion, dehydration, migraine, AMS/HACE, head injury, meningitis, malaria, tension in the neck muscles. At altitude, assume the cause of a severe headache is HACE until proven otherwise. In a malarial area, assume it is malaria until proven otherwise.

Treatment
If you can work out the cause, treat it. Otherwise, give paracetamol for the headache and repeat your secondary survey regularly, including vital signs (especially temperature by thermometer, and tests for HACE if above 2500m).

Migraine
A migraine is a severe headache that usually lasts several hours. The victim is often a regular sufferer and will be able to tell you if this feels like their 'usual migraine' or not. The pain is made worse by strong light and movement, and is often accompanied by nausea, vomiting and sometimes visual changes. If migraine occurs at altitude, check for HACE; note that there is no ataxia or reduced level of consciousness in migraine. If there is even the slightest doubt, treat as HACE and descend.

Treatment
- Rest, lying still with closed eyes in a quiet place and give painkillers (paracetamol or ibuprofen or one 900mg dose of aspirin); give antivomiting medication if needed.
- At altitude migraine may be difficult to tell from early HACE; if in doubt treat for both.

Heart and circulation (vascular) problems

Angina
This is a pain due to narrowed arteries (blood vessels) in the heart muscle, which restricts circulation and oxygen delivery. Brought on by exercise, especially in cold, windy weather, it eases off with rest and treatment. The victim will probably know, 'It's my angina', and be carrying specific medication.

Symptoms and signs

- Typically there is a sudden onset of crushing central chest pain that feels like a tight band or a heavy weight. This may vary from very severe to mild. The pain may travel into the jaw, arm and shoulder (especially the left side), or the upper abdomen (where it can be mistaken for indigestion).
- The pain usually lasts less than 20 minutes. If it lasts longer, it is probably a heart attack.

Treatment

- Lie the victim down (unless they feel better with their head and chest propped up a little or sitting up). They should not walk or stand up. Give an antacid, as indigestion causes similar symptoms.
- Give the victim angina medication (vasodilator medicine such as glyceryl trinitrate (GTN) (or similar). This is a spray or tablet; both are used under the tongue. Do not handle tablets or put spray on hands, as medication is easily absorbed. GTN may cause a severe throbbing headache – an unpleasant but not dangerous side effect. Repeat every 5 minutes, up to three times. If not better after that, assume it is a heart attack.
- Give an aspirin tablet (300mg, preferably crushed and dissolved in water) as soon as possible, then one daily.

Heart attack

This is a serious condition where the heart muscle is damaged due to a complete blockage of the blood vessels that supply it with oxygen. It may occur without warning, while exercising or at rest. The victim may die at any time.

Symptoms and signs

- There is pain as described for angina (above); but there may be no pain at all.
- The pain may last longer than 30 minutes; unlike angina, the pain is not usually helped by angina medication.
- Difficulty breathing, nausea or vomiting and symptoms and signs of shock may occur.

Treatment

- Treat as for angina, giving aspirin and GTN if they are not shocked.
- Manage shock, but do NOT elevate the legs.
- Give oxygen (8 to 10L/min) and be prepared to give BLS.
- Evacuate.

PART 3: Problems and their treatment

Deep vein thrombosis (DVT) and pulmonary embolus (PE)

Clots form in the deep veins of the legs (usually the calves) or lower body (DVT), and can break off (an embolus) and be carried to the lungs, thus blocking their blood vessels (PE).

Symptoms and signs

- DVT: there may be no signs, or a leg may become swollen, painful and tender.
- PE: there may be sudden chest pain, breathlessness, cough with or without blood; collapse and death may occur if an embolus blocks off a substantial section of the lungs.

Treatment

- Rehydrate and give aspirin as for angina.
- DVT: bandage the leg reasonably firmly with a compression bandage from the toes to above the knee, and encourage only gentle ankle and foot movement; gentle, steady walking without a load is OK. Evacuate.
- PE: give oxygen (6 to 10L/min) and evacuate.

Stroke

This is damage to part of the brain caused by a blood clot or a bleed. Factors that predispose to stroke include being over 50 years old, high blood pressure, diabetes, smoking, immobility, the oral contraceptive pill and dehydration.

Symptoms and signs

These may come on suddenly or slowly, over hours or days. It is usually painless.

- Paralysis/weakness of the face, arm or leg
- Speech may be lost or slurred
- Possible vertigo, dizziness, vomiting
- May be unconsciousness or semi-consciousness, but the victim may be fully aware and have some or full understanding of what is being said
- There may be loss of control over, or failure to pass, urine or stools

Treatment

- BLS, shock prevention, monitor vital signs, give oxygen (2 to 4L/min). Nurse in safe airway position, paralysed side down; if unconsciousness is prolonged alternate sides hourly to avoid pressure sores.

- Rest for a day or two, then start moving paralysed limbs.
- Even if unresponsive, talk to them, explaining what is happening, as they may understand.

Haemorrhoids (piles)

Symptoms and signs
- One or more itchy and/or painful lumps may be felt, or seen, at the anus
- There may be bright red blood, often on the toilet paper

Treatment
- Prevent or treat constipation and treat any cough that could make the condition worse.
- Use haemorrhoid suppositories or haemorrhoid ointment to treat the irritation, itchiness or discomfort.
- Any piles that drop out of the anus during a bowel motion should be pushed back inside.
- If the piles become very painful, swollen and red/purple, lay the victim face down and apply occasional cold compresses to the piles, for 3–5 days.

Mental problems

Psychological problems may be caused or aggravated by being a long way from home in strange surroundings, illness or loneliness. Do a thorough secondary survey. Ask about recreational drugs or medication (eg codeine, mefloquine and other medications that can cause mental disturbances).

Critical incident stress
People witnessing, or involved in, serious accidents or deaths may suffer from anxiety, insomnia, flashbacks, guilt, grief or depression (if these symptoms persist, it is called **PTSD (Post Traumatic Stress Disorder)**. If a serious accident or a death occurs, the survivors should be given time to talk about how they are coping, either in a group or individually. If a death is involved (see 'In case of death', p. 81), time should be taken to work through everyone's emotions (anger, guilt, blame) and, if appropriate, organize a ceremony. The people in the group who want to carry on are usually less affected by a major incident than those who want to go home.

PART 3: Problems and their treatment

First aiders/rescuers are likely to feel guilty if the victim dies. You may not always be able to save a life or perform a perfect treatment, but accept that you have done the best you could under the circumstances.

Treatment
As for PUTA (Psychologically Unfit to Travel Abroad) below.

Panic attack
A panic attack usually comes on suddenly and can look like asthma, heart attack, HAPE, or many other conditions..

Symptoms and signs
- Over-breathing, rapid deep breathing, panic and anxiety, feeling afraid
- Tingling in the hands or lips, and cramps of the hands (especially) and feet
- The victim will sometimes tell you 'I am having a panic attack'

Treatment
- Give reassurance while doing a secondary survey, and ask about previous similar attacks.
- Once you are sure of your diagnosis, explain that the fear and anxiety cause over-breathing, which produces more symptoms: calm the victim and their breathing.
- Encourage them to breathe in and out of a paper or plastic bag if cramps are a problem: this re-breathing of exhaled air corrects the developing chemical imbalance that is causing the physical symptoms.

Psychosis
In a psychotic event the victim has no insight into their problem. It may be a first time occurrence or an episode of an existing problem (**bipolar disorder** and **schizophrenia** are common). The victim is not open to reason and may behave in a totally unexpected and dangerous manner (to themselves or others). This is one of the most confronting problems to deal with in a wilderness situation.

Symptoms and signs
Depending on the cause, symptoms may include:
- bizarre, mad behaviour, being on a 'high'; hallucinations (hearing or seeing imaginary things); disorientation, agitation or aggression (beware, the victim can be exceptionally strong while psychotic!)

- paranoia, fear, suspicion; victim cannot be reasoned with, is talking non-stop, or is completely withdrawn.

Treatment
- Assume a non-confrontational manner, take your time over a secondary survey, checking for underlying illness (eg fever, drug abuse, previous history, medication such as mefloquine). Discretely check their clothing and luggage for antipsychotic medication they might have stopped taking.
- Get to a doctor with the necessary medication (eg haloperidol and/or diazepam).
- Prochlorperazine (Stemetil™) (10mg 8 to 12-hourly) OR promethazine 12.5mg can help with anxiety/agitation.
- Evacuate. Be prepared to use physical restraints, especially in aircraft and vehicles, if the victim is a danger to self or pilot/driver. Be prepared for 24 hour/day caring.

'PUTA' (Psychologically Unfit to Travel Abroad)
Typically this occurs in normal healthy, usually first-timers or young travellers a long way from home in a strange country. It is diagnosed after excluding all other possibilities. Unlike psychotics, they can be reasoned with.

Symptoms and signs
- Anxiety, fear, depression; over-worry about health, insomnia, panic attack
- Over-talkative, or silent and withdrawn

Treatment
- Give reassurance, calm them by talking, listening and responding to their concerns: take your time.
- Advise them to rest and do simple, normal tasks (eg washing their clothes, cooking, washing hair).
- Encourage them to look for companionship, to look on the bright side and to stop recreational drugs including alcohol; check for and treat insomnia (below).
- If they are not improving, the 'cure' is to advise them to return to civilisation/home, but make sure they can do so safely.

Insomnia (cannot sleep, poor sleep)

Treatment
- Always check for, and treat, any causes for poor sleep, such as itching, anxiety, cold or discomfort. Improve mattress and warmth.
- Avoid drinking caffeine or alcohol.
- Take time to talk to the person to see if they are anxious; with reassurance, a normal sleep pattern will often establish itself after a few days.
- At altitude, periodic breathing (see p. 166) may disturb sleep and is treated with acetazolamide (Diamox™), the 'high altitude sleeping pill'.
- If all else fails try a sleeping pill for a couple of nights; promethazine (Phenergan™) can be used as a sleeping pill but is very sedative with a 'hangover' the next day.

Note: sleeping pills (and sedatives/antihistamines) should only be used when really necessary as they may cause drowsiness the next day, with possible problems on steep trails and in other sports requiring high concentration and skill levels.

Various other problems

Allergy
This is an overreaction of the immune system to something it perceives as a threat. This reaction may be in response to eating a specific food, taking a medication (see 'Side effects and allergic reactions' p. 37), being in contact with a chemical, pollen, a sting or by application of something to the skin (eg iodine, Band-Aid™, sunscreen, insect repellent). Nasty plants (see p. 131) are a potent source of skin allergy.

Symptoms and signs
May include any of these:
- itchy, red and lumpy skin; this rash may be dry or wet, there may be blisters filled with clear fluid
- swelling, which may be local or general or may affect lips, eyelids, mouth and breathing
- sneezing, headache, dizziness, nausea, vomiting, diarrhoea
- possible anaphylactic shock.

Treatment
- If you can work out the cause, remove it (eg stop the medication, take off the Band-Aid™).
- Give a non-sedating antihistamine (if severe, use promethazine), apply calamine or hydrocortisone cream 8-hourly to rashes.
- In severe cases oral cortisone may be needed.
- Hay fever will need an antihistamine and/or steroid nasal spray.
- Avoid scratching by using cold compresses and covering the area with a light dressing.
- If there is a history of anaphylaxis, or it starts to occur, administer adrenaline and apply a PIB: see 'Anaphylactic shock', p. 67.

Diabetes
Diabetics produce little or no insulin and control their blood sugar level using diet and/or medication (tablets or injections). They often wear a medic-alert tag and carry a glucometer to test their blood sugar level.

Diabetics are more prone to infection, and have poorer circulation and sensation in their limbs (eg they may not feel blisters). As they get fit, lose weight and exercise more, they often need less insulin and will be at increased risk of hypoglycaemia (low blood sugar), so they may have to reduce their medication as they get fit for a trip. Loss of appetite or vomiting (due to illness, altitude, seasickness etc) requires urgent treatment and careful attention to food and liquids, and close monitoring of blood sugar level/medication dose.

There are two kinds of diabetic emergency:

- **HYPOglycaemia** occurs when the blood sugar level drops too LOW (blood sugar values less than 4.0mmol/l). This is caused by too much insulin being administered, not enough food being eaten or too much exercise performed. It is much more common than hyperglycaemia.

- **HYPERglycaemia** is when the blood sugar has gone too HIGH. This is caused by not enough insulin being administered, too much sugary food being eaten, infection or not enough exercise undertaken.

Note: if you cannot decide whether it is hypoglycaemia or hyperglycaemia, treat as hypoglycaemia as this is a more common and more dangerous condition.

Hypoglycaemia

Symptoms and signs

Hypoglycaemia may come on very quickly. Symptoms include:

- tiredness, weakness, sweating, trembling, palpitations; the victim looks pale
- hunger; pins and needles around the mouth
- irritability, emotional swings, verbal/physical aggression, behaving like a drunk
- disorientation, confusion and unconsciousness: death may occur if not treated.

Treatment

- Use the victim's glucometer to confirm the low blood sugar, but don't delay treatment if they are losing consciousness.
- If the victim can swallow safely, give them one of the following as quickly as possible: glucose tablets or syrup (GSF-Syrup™/Hypo-Fit™); a sweet drink (1 cup of water with 4 heaped teaspoon of sugar), a sweet or lolly (not sugar free!), a piece of fruit, or 50–100ml of soft drink (eg lucozade – not a sugarless diet variety!).
- If the victim is unconscious or semiconscious:
  - ▸ place a small amount of glucose tablet or gel, sugar or honey under their tongue and repeat until they revive enough to swallow, and repeat after 10 to 15 minutes if necessary; OR
  - ▸ use an enema to give a sugar solution (4 heaped teaspoons of sugar in 200ml of water), and repeat after 10 to 15 minutes if necessary; OR
  - ▸ if trained, give 1mg of glucagon IM injection.

Note: giving insulin to a HYPOglycaemic victim will kill them!

Hyperglycaemia

Symptoms and signs

It may be difficult to diagnose hyperglycaemia. It comes on slowly and gradually, and may result from another illness (eg flu).

- Victim usually passes a lot of urine, and is thirsty and dehydrated
- Headache, weak, dizzy, nauseous
- Rapid pulse and rapid deep breathing
- Possibly wild and aggressive behaviour

- Victim gradually becoming unconscious with breath smelling of almonds (**ketoacidosis**).

Treatment
- Evacuate urgently for medical treatment.
- Treatment relies on replacing liquids and managing their insulin doses according to their blood sugar test results. Aim for a blood sugar between 8 and 12mmol/L before eating: this is a little higher than normal, but safer in the short term.
- Monitor vital signs.

Seizures, fits, epilepsy
There are several causes of fits. Epilepsy is a common one and the sufferer will usually be on medication to control it. An epileptic fit may be triggered by recently changed/missed medication, or by taking other medication that reduces the effectiveness of the anti-epileptic medication (eg ciprofloxacin, mefloquine, Stemetil™).

Other causes of fits include stress, head injury, alcohol/drug abuse (or withdrawal) or infection (meningitis).

Symptoms and signs
A 'fit' (seizure) consists of:
- sudden loss of consciousness, with wild movements of the arms and legs and clenched teeth
- loss of control over bowel or bladder may occur
- victim is confused, forgetful, weak and dizzy for some time (hours) after the fit has ended.

Treatment
- Keep the victim (and yourself) safe and prevent injury. Do not restrain the victim or put anything in their mouth, but prevent their face from rubbing on the ground.
- Place the victim in the safe airway position (Fig 2.1) when the fit finishes (usually after a few minutes). Do a full secondary survey.
- If the fitting does not stop after 5 minutes, give diazepam (Valium™) up to 10mg by IM injection or rectally (as rectal tubes or enema).
- Evacuate if there are major injuries, the victim is not coping, there are repeated fits, or it is a first-time fit.

Fever of unknown cause

Fever is the body's response to infection or inflammation. There are many possible causes of fever, eg respiratory infections, infectious diseases (including malaria), some abdominal infections or septicaemia. HAPE may cause a non-infective fever up to 38.5°C.

It can be very difficult to identify the cause. Complete a secondary survey, check for rashes, and repeat if necessary. Record the temperature at regular intervals.

If the victim is seriously ill with a high fever and the cause is unknown, consider giving antibiotics as for septicaemia (Appendix 2).

Note: do not lower a fever unnecessarily with paracetamol or NSAIDs.

APPENDICES

APPENDIX 1: CHART OF MEDICATIONS

Caution: the information in this chart is incomplete, so consult your pharmacist or doctor for full information on the medications you are including in your first aid kit.

A * is an indication to refer to the appropriate part of the text for further information on dose.

Generic name (trade name™)	Uses	Dose (adult) (* refer to text)	Remarks, warnings and side effects
ALLERGY, INFLAMMATION AND ITCHING			
• antihistamines: *sedating*: chlorphenamine (Piriton™), promethazine (Phenargan™) *non-sedating*: desloratidine (Neoclarityn™), cetirizine, fexofenidine (Telfast™)	Allergic rashes, itchy skin/ bites, hay fever, prickly heat, anaphylaxis. Sedating form used for insomnia	Follow instructions on packet	Side effects: headache, dry mouth, blurred vision, slow reflexes. Avoid alcohol, avoid in pregnancy. The sedating form especially may cause drowsiness, depress breathing (caution/avoid at altitude)
• hydrocortisone cream 1% (Hydrocort™)	Rashes, allergies, bites, mild sunburn, piles	Apply directly 8-hourly	External use only. Not to be used on infected or broken skin
• prednisolone 10mg	Severe allergy, asthma attack, anaphylactic shock	*	Takes 4–6 hours to start working. Given for short term only
ALTITUDE ILLNESS (AMS, HACE AND HAPE)			
• acetazolamide (Diamox™)	AMS prevention, AMS and HACE treatment. Periodic breathing/poor sleep at altitude	*	Takes 12 hours to fully start working. For more info and side effects, see p. 39. Avoid in severe sulfa allergy, pregnancy, diabetes, kidney disease

Generic name (trade name™)	Uses	Dose (adult) (* refer to text)	Remarks, warnings and side effects
• dexamethasone	HACE/severe AMS, asthma, anaphylactic shock	*	Give the last 3 doses 12-hourly. Multiple side effects with longer use of the medication. More information p. 171
• nifedipine modified release (MR) or long acting (LA) /Adalat LA™, Adipine MR™, Coroday MR™)	HAPE	*	Side effects: sudden fall in blood pressure, fainting, dizziness, flushing, headache. More information p. 173
ANTIBIOTICS – SEE APPENDIX 2			
ANTIVOMITING AND ANTINAUSEA			
• prochlorperazine (Stemetil™) 5mg tab	a) Nausea/vomiting, may be used for acute vertigo see viral labyrinthitis, p. 154	5–10mg 8-hourly. Use only for 2 or 3 days	Side effects: severe spasms of neck, face and eye muscles especially in younger people (antidotes: cogentin or diphenhydramine). Avoid in pregnancy, children, epilepsy. May depress breathing, cause drowsiness, dry mouth, drop blood pressure, photosensitivity
	b) May be useful for acute anxiety, agitation in psychosis	5–10mg 8 to 12-hourly	As above but risks of severe spasms is higher owing to increased dose and duration of treatment
• prochlorperazine (Buccastem™) 3mg buccal (inside gum)	Nausea/vomiting	1–2 tabs 12-hourly	Buccal tablets are placed high on the gum behind the upper lip and allowed to dissolve

APPENDICES

Generic name (trade name™)	Uses	Dose (adult) (* refer to text)	Remarks, warnings and side effects
ANTIVOMITING AND ANTINAUSEA (continued)			
• promethazine (Phenargan™) 25mg tab and suppository	As for Stemetil™, especially for seasickness	*	As for Stemetil™, especially drowsiness
• ondansetron wafers (Zofran Zydis™)	Nausea/vomiting	1 wafer 12-hourly	Wafers are placed on tongue, allowed to dissolve, then swallowed. Side effects similar to Stemetil™. Avoid taking with azithromycin
CONSTIPATION			
laxative tablets (Bisacodyl™)	Constipation	1–2 tabs at night	May cause griping belly pain. Increase fibre/ liquid intake. Avoid under 12 years old. Avoid if intestinal obstruction is suspected
DIARRHOEA (SEE ALSO ANTIBIOTICS APPENDIX 2)			
• loperamide (Imodium™)	To slow down diarrhoea	2 caps, then one after each loose stool (max 8 caps per day)	Don't stop the diarrhoea, just slow it down. Side effects: dry mouth, blurred vision. Avoid under 9 years old. Avoid if bloody diarrhoea
DISINFECTANT			
• burn cream: silver sulfadiazine	Infected burns	See burns	External use only. Avoid in sulfa allergy

Generic name (trade name™)	Uses	Dose (adult) (* refer to text)	Remarks, warnings and side effects
• povi-iodine (Savlon™, Betadine™)	a) General disinfectant, wound cleaning	1 tablespoon in 250ml water	External use only, skin allergy
	b) Disinfection of instruments	1 tablespoon in 100ml water	Leave 10 minutes
• Chlorine tabs (NaDCC) or household bleach (hypochlorite solution)	Water disinfection	*	Use only unscented household bleach with no detergent or soap. Bleach loses its potency after 6 months of being opened
• Chlorhexidine	Disinfection of skin and dental cavities; mouthwash	*	
EYE AND EAR			
• antibiotic ointment for eyes: chloramphenicol	Eye infection, abrasion, superficial foreign object	*	Side effects: local allergic reaction, stop if symptoms get worse
• anti-inflammatory/ antibiotic drops for ears (Sofradex H.C™)	Infection or inflammation of external ear canal	*	Store cool, as heat sensitive. Side effects: local allergic reaction, stop if symptoms get worse
• anaesthetic eye drops: tetracaine (Minims- Amethocaine™)	Snow blindness, removing foreign object etc	*	Effect lasts for up to 4 hours. Once anaesthetized, the eye is best padded shut until sensitive again (to avoid further injury)
INDIGESTION			
• simple antacids (Gaviscon™, Gelusil™ etc)	Heartburn, indigestion	*	Best not taken with other medications as may reduce their absorption

Generic name (trade name™)	Uses	Dose (adult) (* refer to text)	Remarks, warnings and side effects
INDIGESTION (continued)			
• Lansoprazole (Prevacid™)	Heartburn, indigestion	30mg twice daily, try stopping after 2 days	Use if simple antacids don't work. Take 30min before food
PAINKILLERS (ANALGESICS) – SEE CHAPTER 4			
• paracetamol (Panadol™)	Mild to moderate aches, pains, flu, headache, fever	1000mg (2 tabs) 4 to 6-hourly. Daily maximum: 4000mg	Remarks and side effects, p. 42
• aspirin	a) Aches and pains, flu, headache, fever, arthritis, inflammation, broken tooth, migraine	300–600mg 4 to 6-hourly. Daily maximum: 3600mg	Side effects: indigestion, retinal bleeding at high altitude. Take with food. Avoid if history of stomach ulcer, stomach bleeding, allergy or asthma. Avoid under 16 years old
	b) Heart attack	300mg daily, until specialist advice	
• ibuprofen (Brufen™)	Mild to moderate pain, pain with inflammation or infection, women's period pains, sprains and strains	200–400mg 6 to 8-hourly. Daily maximum: 2400mg	Take with food. Remarks and side effects (p. 43) and see naproxen below. Not recommended above 5000m

Generic name (trade name™)	Uses	Dose (adult) (* refer to text)	Remarks, warnings and side effects
• naproxen (Naprosyn™) 250mg	Moderate pain, trekker's knee, muscle, bone and joint pain, pain due to trauma, dental pain, acute gout, kidney stones	1 tab 6 to 8-hourly. Daily maximum: 1000mg	An NSAID. Avoid in asthma, indigestion, the elderly, pregnancy, breastfeeding, kidney disease; do NOT use with other NSAIDs; give with food
• diclofenac (Voltarol™) 50mg suppository	Severe pain. Same indications as naproxen.	1–2 suppositories 8 to 12-hourly	Same as naproxen
• codeine phosphate	a) Moderate pain	*	See p. 44.
	b) Cough, diarrhoea	15–30mg 8 to12-hourly	Mild cough suppressant, slows diarrhoea
• tramadol 50mg (Zamadol™, Zydol™)	Moderate to severe pain	50–100mg 4-hourly. Max dose 400mg in 24 hours	Similar to codeine consider giving with an antivomiting medication
• morphine	Severe pain, eg broken bones, burns, heart attack	5–10mg by IM or SC injection every 4 hours	Side effects: depresses breathing (antidote: Narcan™), hallucinations. Avoid in asthma attack and altitude illness. Caution at altitude. Side effects as for codeine

Generic name (trade name™)	Uses	Dose (adult) (* refer to text)	Remarks, warnings and side effects
PAINKILLERS (ANALGESICS) (continued)			
• fentanyl lozenge 'lolly' (Actiq™) 800 micrograms	Severe pain, eg broken bones, burns, dislocations	one application over a 15-minute period, repeat after 30 minutes if needed. Maximum of four dose units daily	Simple to use, effective and rapid onset; see p. 44. Controlled drug, off label use
• methoxyflurane (Penthrox™)	Inhaled instant short-term relief of moderate to severe pain	*	Avoid overdose, use in confined spaces may affect carers, see p. 45
RESPIRATORY AND OTHER PROBLEMS			
• asthma spray (reliever) salbutamol (Ventolin™) spray is coloured blue	a) Asthma	*	To increase effectiveness, use a spacer (see Fig 21.1). Keep spray warm in very cold conditions. Side effects: palpitations, tremors
	b) May be helpful for anaphylactic shock	*	

Generic name (trade name™)	Uses	Dose (adult) (* refer to text)	Remarks, warnings and side effects
• flu and sinus medication	Flu, head cold, nasal congestion	Refer to packet	Side effects: drowsiness, may depress breathing (caution at altitude). These medications often contain painkillers. Avoid: alcohol, blood pressure and antidepressant medication
• glyceryl trinitrate (GTN) spray	a) angina b) heart attack	*	Side effects include headache and low blood pressure. Flammable/explosive near flames. Caution with Viagra™ and other similar drugs
• phenylephrine or pseudoephedrine nasal drops or spray	a) Nasal congestion, sinusitis, earache b) May be useful for: anaphylactic shock, nosebleed	3–4 drops or one spray 6 to 8-hourly into nostril *	Insert drops with head upside down, or right back and to one side. Maximum 5 days' treatment. Side effects: increased blood pressure, palpitations, can destabilize diabetes or glaucoma. Avoid in pregnancy.
• prednisolone	a) Severe asthma attack b) Anaphylactic shock	*	Takes 3–4 hours to work. A lifesaving drug in severe asthma attack. Used in anaphylactic shock to prevent relapse. Many serious side effects: indigestion, nausea, suppresses healing, thrush, depression, psychosis, insomnia (it is generally safe for short term use).

APPENDIX 2: ANTIBIOTICS

The alphabetic list below sets out the antibiotics recommended for various problems mentioned in the book. Before giving an antibiotic you must read the reference in the text.

See also Chapter 3.

Warning:

- Antibiotics are prescription-only medications and they should only be given by appropriately trained persons. See 'Prescription-only medications', p. 35.
- As antibiotic resistance occurs, the advice below may become outdated. If this book is more than three years old, check this appendix with your doctor.
- If there is a severe allergy (especially an anaphylactic reaction) to any antibiotic, such as penicillin, this must be identified before departure and alternatives provided. See 'Side effects and allergic reactions', p.37.
- The penicillin antibiotics are co-amoxiclav, amoxicillin and flucloxacillin. Alternatives are mentioned in the text below. Do not give cefalexin to people with penicillin anaphylaxis.
- Norfloxacin is an alternative to ciprofloxacin. Tinidazole is an alternative to metronidazole. See 'Remarks, warnings and side effects' below.

Dose and duration

Animal bites

- co-amoxiclav (625mg 8-hourly) for 5 days
- if severe or getting worse, add metronidazole (400mg 8-hourly); give both antibiotics for 7 days.
- if penicillin allergic, replace co-amoxiclav with clarithromycin (500mg 12-hourly).

Appendicitis

- co-amoxiclav (625mg 8-hourly) for 10 days
- OR cefalexin (500mg 6-hourly) PLUS metronidazole (400mg 6-hourly) for 10 days
- cefalexin may be replaced by amoxicillin (1000mg 6-hourly)

Bacterial vaginosis
- metronidazole (400mg 12-hourly) for 7 days

Bronchitis, sinusitis
- amoxicillin (500mg 6-hourly) OR, if penicillin allergic, clarithromycin (500mg 12-hourly) for 7–10 days (sinusitis) or 5 days (bronchitis)

Chlamydia
- azithromycin (1000mg once only) OR clarithromycin (500mg 12-hourly for 7 days)

Cystitis
- cefalexin (500mg 12-hourly) OR amoxicillin (500mg 8-hourly) for 3 days in women, 7 days in men
- if no improvement after a day or two, change to co-amoxiclav (625mg 8-hourly)

Diarrhoea – amoebic
- metronidazole (800mg 8-hourly for 5–10 days) OR tinidazole (2000mg given as one daily dose for 3 days)

Diarrhoea – bacterial
- ciprofloxacin (1000mg taken once; if improving but not completely settled after 12 hours, continue with 500mg 12-hourly for 2–3 days)
- if there is no improvement after 12 hours of the first ciprofloxacin dose, stop the ciprofloxacin and change to azithromycin (500mg daily for 3 days)
- ciprofloxacin may be replaced by norfloxacin (800mg once, then 400mg 12-hourly)

Note: if there is no improvement after 48 hours, refer to the 'Antibiotic protocol for severe diarrhoea of unknown cause', p. 151.

Diarrhoea – cyclospora
- co-trimoxazole (one tab 12-hourly) for 7 days

Diarrhoea – giardia
- metronidazole (400mg 8-hourly for 5 days) OR tinidazole (2000mg given as a single dose, repeated on day 3)

Ear infection – middle
- amoxicillin (500mg 8-hourly) for 5 days OR clarithromycin (500mg 12-hourly)

Ear infection – outer
- simple infection: Sofradex HC™ drops
- severe infection: flucloxacillin (250mg 6-hourly) OR co-amoxiclav (375mg 6-hourly) OR ciprofloxacin (500mg 12-hourly) for 5 days

Eye – orbital cellulitis
- co-amoxiclav (625mg 8-hourly) for 7 days
- OR amoxicillin (500mg 6-hourly) PLUS flucloxacillin (250mg 6-hourly) for 7 days
- OR, if penicillin allergic, azithromycin (500mg daily) PLUS ciprofloxacin (500mg twice daily) for 7 days

Gonorrhoea
- azithromycin (2000mg) PLUS ciprofloxacin (500mg once only OR 400mg IM if available)

Impetigo
- flucloxacillin (500mg 6-hourly) for 5 days OR, if penicillin allergic, clarithromycin (500mg 12-hourly)

Kidney infection
- ciprofloxacin (500mg 12-hourly) for 7 days

Meningitis
- co-amoxiclav (625mg 6-hourly) for 7–10 days PLUS (if the victim is not having fits) ciprofloxacin (500mg 12-hourly)
- co-amoxiclav may be replaced by amoxicillin (1000mg 6-hourly)

Mouth infections
- if not involving a large area of the gums, treat as for 'tooth abscess'. If involving a large area of the gum, give metronidazole (400mg 8-hourly) for 5 days
- give dexamethasone at the same time as antibiotics at the HACE dose (p. 172) for 4 days
- if not improving, add co-amoxiclav (625mg 8-hourly) for 5 days

A diagnosis of AMS is based on:

- a rise in altitude within the last 3 days
- presence of a headache (usually), plus at least one other symptom
- a total score of 3 or more from the questions below.

A score of 3 to 5 indicates mild AMS (with all symptoms mild in nature). A score of 6 or more indicates moderate to severe AMS (with some or all symptoms severe in nature). In this case check for HACE.

Add together the individual scores for each symptom to get the *total score*.

Headache	No headache	0
	Mild headache	1
	Moderate headache	2
	Severe headache, incapacitating	3
Gastrointestinal symptoms	None	0
	Poor appetite or nausea	1
	Moderate nausea and/or vomiting	2
	Severe nausea and/or vomiting	3
Fatigue and/or weakness	Not tired or weak	0
	Mild fatigue/weakness	1
	Moderate fatigue/weakness	2
	Severe fatigue/weakness	3
Dizziness/light-headedness	Not dizzy	0
	Mild dizziness	1
	Moderate dizziness	2
	Severe dizziness, incapacitating	3
Difficulty sleeping	Slept as well as usual	0
	Did not sleep as well as usual	1
	Woke many times, poor sleep	2
	Could not sleep at all	3
Total score		

The Children's Lake Louise Score (CLLS) can be downloaded from www.adventuremedicalconsulting.co.uk/page/99/Medical-Forms.htm

APPENDIX 7: MARINE BITES AND STINGS

© Dr Edi Albert and Adventure Medic 2016
With thanks to Dr Peter Fenner

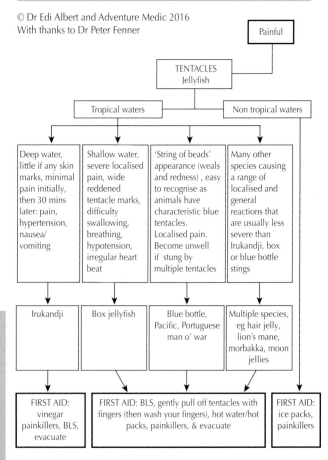

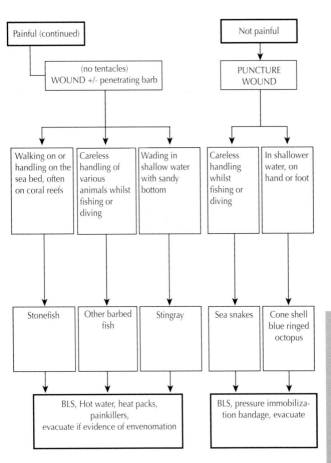

APPENDIX 8: THE SKELETON AND INTERNAL ORGANS

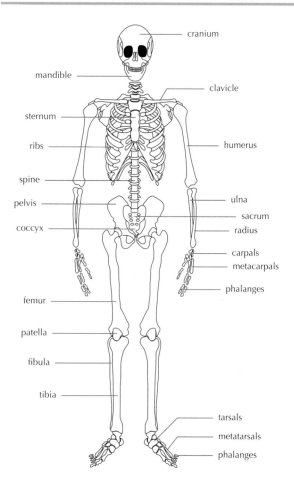

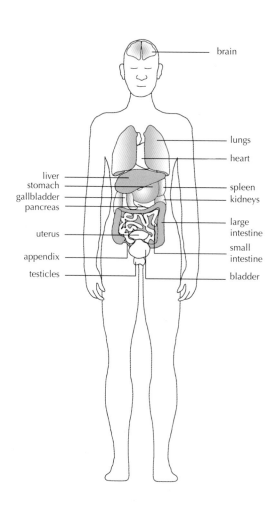

APPENDIX 9: FIRST AID KITS

The first aid kits listed here are suggestions only: adjust them according to your needs. Kit preparation depends on the area to be visited, the season, number of people in the group (including local staff and porters) and their age/fitness levels, the activities to be undertaken and duration of the trip, degree of remoteness and the availability of rescue and medical facilities. It will also depend on which advanced procedures you are able to perform eg stitching wounds, giving injections.

Consider these points:

- divide your kit into containers of appropriate categories: medications, trauma & dressings, instruments etc; prepare a separate 'grab bag' for minor trauma
- containers must be waterproof, lockable, light coloured (darker colours cause excess heating): keep out of direct sunlight and prevent freezing
- accessibility of contents: lids marked with contents, individual items packed in clear plastic bags or containers
- checklist of contents, notebook, pen, incident forms, controlled medications documents, head torch, batteries, a small mirror, and a satellite phone with relevant phone numbers and plenty of credit.

Personal medications for pre-existing illnesses, and alternatives due to allergy to certain medications, are the responsibility of the individual. Each participant should bring and carry Band-Aids™, a crepe bandage, antiseptic wipes, blister patches, paracetamol, antacid, water disinfectant tablets, hand sanitizer, insect repellent and sunblock.

Most items mentioned are available in most developing countries (common exceptions: Steristrips™, Moleskin™, prochlorperazine (Stemetil™ suppositories, Buccastem™), methoxyflurane (Penthrox™), SAM splint™, Ziploc™ bags.

- ***First aid kit no 1*** is for a large group (eg 10 to 15 people with cooking staff and porters, for a trip up to one month) or for a base camp.

- ***First aid kit no 2*** is for a small group (eg 6 people on a one-week trip) or for a field kit.

- ***First aid kit no 3*** is for two travellers in a developing country.

	1) large group	2) small group	3) two people
Instruments			
thermometer	1	1	1
tweezers – fine point and toothed	2	2	1
scissors, sharp: one fine, one large	one of each	one of each	1 fine
ordinary sewing needles	1 pkt	1 pkt	1 pkt
safety pins	5	3	2
forceps (artery)	2	1	
scalpel with various blades	1	1	
disposable razors	1 packet		
syringe 20ml or bigger	1	1	
syringe 10ml (and needles)	1	1	1
syringe 2ml (and needles)	10	2	1
protective gloves	10 pairs	5 pairs	1 pair
rubber gloves (washing-up)	2 pairs	1	
enema tube	1	1	
sharps container	1		
Dressings and wound care			
Band-Aids™	60	20	10
blister dressing (Moleskin™)	3 packets	1 packet	1 packet
cotton buds	1 packet	1 packet	
gauze squares 5cm	30	10	5
sterile non-stick dressings 10cm (eg Melolin™)	30	10	2
large wound dressing	2	1	
sanitary pads (for absorbent padding)	10	5	1
plastic food wrap (Clingwrap™, Saranwrap™)	1 roll	1 roll	
adhesive tape bandage 10cm, 2.5cm	1 roll of each	1 roll of 2.5cm	
triangular bandages	2	1	
cotton bandages 10cm x 1.5m	10	2	1
elastic bandages 10/15cm	5	2	2
crepe bandages 10cm x 1.5m	5	1	1

APPENDICES

	1) large group	2) small group	3) two people
nasal tampons	1pkt		
duct tape	2 rolls	1 roll	1 roll
closures (Steristrips™) 6mm	4 packets	1 packet	1 packet
tincture of benzoin (prone to leaks: double wrap!)	small bottle		
alcohol swabs	box 100	50	20
petroleum jelly (Vaseline™)	1 tube/jar	1 small tube/jar	
SAM splint™ (large)	2	2	
eye pads	2	2	
Medications			
Allergy, inflammation and itch			
antihistamine tablets (sedating)	20 tabs	10 tabs	10 tabs
antihistamine tables (non-sedating) cetirizine, desloratidine or fexofenadine	30	20	10
promethazine 25mg	10	5	
promethazine suppository 12.5mg	5		
anti-inflammatory cream/ointment/gel	1 tube	1 tube	
hydrocortisone cream 1%	15g tube	15g tube	15g tube
calamine or Eurax™ cream	15g tube	15g tube	15g tube
insect repellent	1	1	
Altitude illness (if sleeping above 2500m)			
acetazolamide 250mg (Diamox™)	100 tabs	20 tabs	20 tabs
nifedipine modified release (MR) or long acting (LA) 20 to 30mg	20 tabs	10 tabs	6 tabs
dexamethasone 4mg	40 tabs	30 tabs	20 tabs
Antibiotics			
ciprofloxacin 500mg or norfloxacin 400mg	40 tabs	20 tabs	10 tabs
co-amoxiclav 250mg	40 tabs	30 tabs	20 tabs
amoxicillin 250mg	30 tabs	20 tabs	20 tabs
cephalexin 250mg	30 tabs	20 tabs	20 tabs
flucloxacillin 500mg	40 tabs	20 tabs	

	1) large group	2) small group	3) two people
clarithromycin 500mg	40 tabs	20 tabs	
doxycycline 100mg (if going to a marine environment or tick-infested area)	20 tabs	10 tabs	
azithromycin 500mg	40 tabs	20 tabs	
metronidazole 400mg or tinidazole 400/500mg	40 tabs	30 tabs	15 tabs
Antibiotic/antifungal skin applications			
antibiotic ointment (mupirocin or fucidin)	15g tube	15g tube	15g tube
antifungal cream (miconazole, clotrimazole, terbinafine)	15g tube	15g tube	
Burn			
burn cream (silver sulfadiazine or Aloe Vera gel)	2 x 20g tubes	1 x 20g tube	
Constipation			
laxative (Bisacodyl™)	20 tabs	10 tabs	
Dental			
clove oil (Dentaik™)	bottle		
temporary filling material (Cavit™ or Dentafix™)	1 tube		
fluoride varnish (Duraphat™)	1 tube		
mouthwash (chlorhexidine)	1 bottle		
tin foil for splints	20cm length		
all the above OR a dental first aid kit (proprietary)	1		
Diarrhoea			
loperamide (Imodium™)	30 caps	15 caps	10 caps
Disinfectant			
povi-iodine (Betadine™) or Savlon™ or Dettol™	bottle	small bottle	small bottle
Dettol™ soap	1	1	
Disinfectant for water			
chlorine tablets (NaDCC) or unscented household bleach	as appropriate	as appropriate	as appropriate

	1) large group	2) small group	3) two people
Eye and ear infection			
antibiotic ointment for eye (chloramphenicol)	1 tube	1 tube	
anti-inflammatory/ antibiotic drops for ear (Sofradex HC™)	1 bottle	1 bottle	
anaesthetic eye drops (tetracaine, Minims Amethocaine™)	4 minims	2 minims	
Haemorrhoid (piles)			
haemorrhoid ointment	1 tube	1 tube	
haemorrhoid suppositories	5		
Indigestion			
antacid simple (Gaviscon™ etc)	40 tabs	20 tabs	
ranitidine 150mg	20 tabs	10 tabs	10 tabs
Nausea and vomiting			
prochlorperazine (as Buccastem™ 3mg buccal tablet or Stemetil™ 5mg tablet)	20	10	5
prochlorperazine (Stemetil™) suppositories or injectable ampoule	5	3	
promethazine (Phenergan™) tablets	20	10	
promethazine (Phenergan™) suppository or injection (for seasickness)	5	3	
ondansetron wafers (Zofran Zydis™)	10		
Painkillers (analgesics)			
paracetamol 500mg	60 tabs	20 tabs	10 tabs
aspirin 300mg	40 tabs		
ibuprofen 400mg	60 tabs/caps	40 tabs/caps	20 tabs/caps
codeine phosphate 30mg*	40 tabs	20 tabs	10 tabs
naproxen (Naproxen™) 250mg tablet	40 tabs	15 tabs	
diclofenac (Voltarol™) 50mg suppository	10	5	
oxycodone 10mg	30 tabs	15 tabs	
methoxyflurane (Penthrox™) inhaler	2	1	

	1) large group	2) small group	3) two people
lidocaine gel	1 tube		
ORS (oral rehydration solution)			
eg Diorylate™, Gastrolyte™, Jeevan Jal™, Electrobion™, Rehidrat™	10 packets	4 packets	2 packets
Respiratory (breathing) problems			
phenylephrine or pseudoephedrine nasal drops/spray	1 bottle/spray	1 bottle/spray	
flu and sinus medication	20 tabs/caps	10 tabs/caps	
throat lozenges	40	15	5
asthma reliever spray (salbutamol)	1	1	
prednisolone 10mg	50 tabs	30 tabs	
tiger balm or eucalyptus oil	1 tube/jar		
Other medication			
diazepam 5mg tablets	20 tabs	10 tabs	
diazepam rectal tubes 5mg	2		
glyceryl trinitrate (GTN) spray or similar	1		
Other items recommended			
hyperbaric bag and/or oxygen (if going above 3000m)	1 bag/cylinder		
face mask for rescue breathing (Laerdal™ mask)	1	1	
Blizzard bag™ or space blanket	1	1	
bivvy/bothy bag	enough for whole group	1	
sunscreen	1 tube	1 tube	
glucose tablets	10		
gas lighter	1	1	
square of boiled clean dry cotton sheet (1 metre)	1	1	
pencil	1	1	
incident forms (sample available from www.adventuremedical consulting.co.uk/page/99/Medical-Forms.htm	5	2	

	1) large group	2) small group	3) two people
DOCTORS, PARAMEDICS OR SPECIFICALLY TRAINED FIRST AIDERS MAY CONSIDER THE FOLLOWING			
oto/opthalmo/stetho-scope	1		
pulse oximeter (oxygen saturation meter)	1		
airways	selection (including nasopharyngeal)		
manual suction device	1		
Ambu bag™	1		
nasogastric tube	1	1	
sutures with needles	various sizes		
lidocaine local anaesthetic injection	5 ampoules	2 ampoules	
IV/IM antibiotics, antiemetic, antipsychotic, dexamethasone, glucagon, diazepam, epinephrine (adrenaline), tetanus booster	as appropriate	as appropriate	
blood volume expanders 500ml infusion bag/giving set	2		
ketamine* anaesthetic for IM or IV injection	5 ampoules		
fluorescein eye stain	2 minims		
morphine for IM injection* and/or fentanyl lozenges*	5 ampoules or lozenges		
naloxone (Narcan™)	2 ampoules		
parecoxib (Dynastat™) for injection	5 ampoules		
anti-psychotic IM and oral			
GROUP LEADER/DOCTOR SHOULD ALSO HAVE READILY AVAILABLE			
Trauma grab bag with two elastic bandages, small bivvy bag, spare fleece or down jacket, whistle and, if appropriate, a radio, mobile and/or satellite telephone.			

* For Customs purposes, carry correct documentation for any controlled drugs and a doctor's letter stating these medications are for expedition use.

APPENDIX 10: USEFUL CONTACTS AND SOURCES OF INFORMATION

Travel Medicine and General Information

- Adventure Medical Consulting (UK)
  www.adventuremedicalconsulting.co.uk
- Immunization information (UK)
  www.fitfortravel.nhs.uk
- Travel Health Pro (UK)
  www.travelhealthpro.org.uk
- WHO – World Health Organization (USA)
  www.who.int
- Medical Advisory Service for Travellers Abroad – MASTA (UK)
  www.masta-travel-health.com
- TMVC – Travellers' Medical and Vaccination Center (Australia)
  www.traveldoctor.com.au
- Travelhealth.co.uk (UK)
  www.travelhealth.co.uk
- CIWEC Clinic Travel Medicine (Nepal)
  https://ciwechospital.com
- Nepal International Clinic – NIC (Nepal)
  www.nepalinternationalclinic.com
- World Extreme Medicine (UK)
  https://worldextrememedicine.com
- International narcotics control board (Austria)
  www.incb.org/incb/en/publications/Guidelines.html
  provides information on customs and legal considerations of medical drugs and international travel
- *Oxford Handbook of Expedition and Wilderness Medicine*, 2nd Edition, ISBN 978-0-19-968841-8. A great comprehensive resource for expedition doctors and leaders

Note: The Covid-19 pandemic is presently severely affecting adventure travel; refer to the numerous sources in Appendix 10 for up-to-date travel information, and the Covid-19 resources on the UIAA website (www.theuiaa.org/covid-19)

Altitude, frostbite
- The British Mountaineering Council (UK)
  www.thebmc.co.uk
- Advice on Altitude Illness
  (International Climbing and Mountaineering Federation)
  www.theuiaa.org/medical_advice.html
- MEDEX (Medical Expeditions UK)
  www.medex.org.uk/medex_book/about_book.php
- Frostbite advice (UK) is available from
  www.christopherimray.co.uk/highaltitudemedicine/
  highaltitudemedicine.htm
  (in a frostbite emergency, you can contact Dr Chris Imray, Surgeon,
  +44 0247 696 4000 chrisimray@aol.com)
- Himalayan Rescue Association – HRA (Nepal)
  www.himalayanrescue.org
- Blizzard Protection Systems (UK)
  www.blizzardsurvival.com

Water
- DDRC on diver health and advice (UK)
  www.ddrc.org/diving
- Divers Alert Network – DAN (international)
  www.dan.org
- International Emergency Hotline
  +1 919 684 9111 (they accept collect calls from anywhere in the
  world, except California)
- The DAN World Diving Emergency Service (DES) Hotline
  http://danap.org/emergency/des_hotline.php
  (Toll Free in Australia) 1800 088 200
  Outside Australia +61 8 8212 9242
- Rescue for River Runners (R3)
  www.rescueforriverrunners.com
- Advice about crocodiles
  https://environment.des.qld.gov.au/wildlife/animals/living-with/
  crocodiles/croc-wise
- Video on how to survive a fall into freezing water
  www.youtube.com/watch?v=Wz3gy5XyaBo

Water disinfection
Advice on water disinfection (International Climbing and Mountaineering Federation) www.theuiaa.org/mountain-medicine/medical-advice/ and follow link to '6. Water disinfection in the mountains'

Poisons, bites and stings
- National Poisons Information Centre (UK)
  www.npis.org
  for information and first aid advice, dial 111
- Queensland Poisons Information (Australia)
  www.qld.gov.au/emergency/safety/poisons.html
  for information and first aid advice, dial 131 126
  (useful for jellyfish and other marine stings/ poisoning – open 24 hours)
- National Capital Poison Center (USA)
  www.poison.org
  for information and first aid advice, call 1 800 222 1222
- 'Australian bites and stings'
  an excellent app for Australia
- Staying safe around bears
  www.nps.gov/subjects/bears/safety.htm

Various
- Methoxyflurane (Penthrox™)
  www.ambulance.qld.gov.au/docs/clinical/dtprotocols/DTP_Methoxyflurane.pdf

INDEX OF DIAGRAMS

INDEX

A

Abdominal (belly)
    problems 153
    thrusts (Heimlich manoeuvre) 61
    wounds 120
Abscess 192
    ear 186
    tooth 188
Accident and illness protocol 48
Acetazolamide 39
Acute mountain sickness (AMS)
    See Altitude illness
Adhesive closures 114
AIDS *See HIV*
Airway (opening the) 53
Allergy
    anaphylactic shock 67
    general 206
    to medications 37
Altitude
    AMS 167
    HACE 167
    HAPE 168
    illness 165
    medications at 38, 171
    prevention at 23
Amoebic diarrhoea 150
Amputation 121
AMS 167
Anaesthetizing (a wound) 111
Anaphylactic shock 67
Angina 200
Animal
    bites 119
    prevention 17
Ankle 103
Appendicitis 156
Assisted breathing 57
Asthma 162
Ataxia (HACE) 167
Avalanche
    hypothermia 137
    rescue 230
    risks 26
AVPU scale 75

B

Back injury 84
Bacterial diarrhoea 149
Bandage
    doughnut (ring pad) 118
    pressure immobilization
        bandage (PIB) 125
Barotrauma 175
Basic Life Support (BLS) 52
Bears 17
Bed bugs 127
Bees 127
Bends (the) 175
Bipolar disorder 204
Bites 124
    prevention 17
Black widow spider *See Spiders*
Bladder
    infection 194
    obstruction (pelvis fracture) 107
Bleeding
    controlling external 58
    deadly (life-threatening) 53, 58
    head injury 86
    heavy menstrual 196
    internal 159
    nosebleed 123
Blepharitis 182
Blindness
    river 19
    snow 185
Blisters 122
Blocked
    airway (choking) 60
    nose (sinusitis) 161
Blood infection/poisoning *See Septicaemia*
Blood pressure (fall in) *See Shock*
BLS (Basic Life Support) 52
Blue bottle jellyfish 230
Blue ringed octopus 128
Boils 192
    gumboil (tooth) 188
    in the ear 186
Bowel
    obstruction 157
    protruding under skin (hernia) 158

245

INDEX

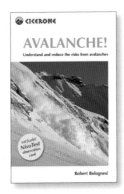
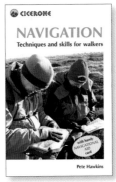
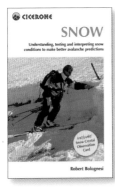
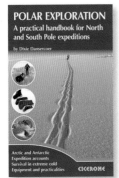
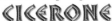

LISTING OF INTERNATIONAL CICERONE GUIDES

CICERONE

Trust Cicerone to guide your next adventure,
wherever it may be around the world...

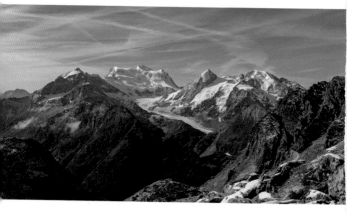

Discover guides for hiking, mountain walking, backpacking,
trekking, trail running, cycling and mountain biking, ski touring,
climbing and scrambling in Britain, Europe and worldwide.

Connect with Cicerone online and find inspiration.

- buy books and ebooks
- articles, advice and trip reports
- podcasts and live events
- GPX files and updates
- regular newsletter

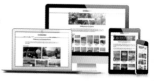

cicerone.co.uk